D1327874

The
Highland
Vet

The
Highland
Vet

A Year at Thurso

Guy Gordon

**EBURY
SPOTLIGHT**

1 3 5 7 9 10 8 6 4 2

Ebury Spotlight, an imprint of Ebury Publishing
20 Vauxhall Bridge Road
London SW1V 2SA

Ebury Spotlight is part of the Penguin Random House group
of companies whose addresses can be found at
global.penguinrandomhouse.com

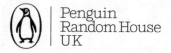

Penguin
Random House
UK

First published by Ebury Spotlight in 2022

www.penguin.co.uk

A CIP catalogue record for this book is available from the British Library

ISBN 9781529148992

Printed and bound in Great Britain by Clays Ltd, Elcograf S.p.A.
Imported into the EEA by Penguin Random House Ireland,
Morrison Chambers, 32 Nassau Street, Dublin D02 YH68.

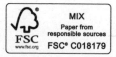

Remembering my dad, Mike Gordon (1946–2020).
He would have loved this book.

Contents

Autumn

Winter

Foreword

As a child in primary school, I had an idea that I wanted to be a vet when I grew up. I loved animals and thought it would be an obvious and simple transition to become one. I embarked upon my training early when, one day, I found a tiny bird alone on the ground. With no visible sign of its parents or nest, I decided to look after the wee orphan myself. I filled a small box with cotton wool and placed it on a hot water bottle. This was to be its new home. I attempted to give it some sustenance with the aid of an eye-drop dispenser containing a variety of foodstuffs I thought might be suitable; bread soaked in warm milk and mushed-up worms. Yuck.

I would like to say that my ministrations proved successful and that the chick thrived and was eventually released successfully back into the wild. But, despite my parents' and my best efforts, the little creature didn't survive. The experience taught me a few things, not least that there was a lot more to this vet business than I had imagined and that perhaps my vocation lay elsewhere.

Another childhood memory I have involving animals had a much more positive outcome. One afternoon, after school, my brother discovered his pet mouse, Sammy, lying comatose in his cage and breathing very weakly. There was much wailing and weeping from us three children until the cavalry arrived in the shape of my father, home from work. He put Sammy in a blanket-lined shoebox and the trusty eye-drop dispenser was pressed into service once again. This time around, it contained a tot of whisky. We carefully placed Sammy and his box beside the fire. By the time we had finished our tea and gone back to check on him, he was scampering all over the living room as if nothing untoward had ever happened. We had Sammy for a good long while after that, thanks to Dad and a wee drop of the good stuff.

In more recent times, my family and I became the proud owners of a dog, my first one ever. And not just any dog. Carlos the lurcher was a prince among hounds, the fastest in any park. We found him at Battersea Dogs Home and what a find he was. The care Carlos was given when he ruptured his cruciate ligament (as a result of running, of course) was exceptional, and made me all the more in awe of veterinary practices. Sadly, Carlos is no longer with us these days, but he lives on in our hearts.

In summary, I have a lot of respect for the vital work that vets do. And so, when I was first asked to narrate the *Highland Vet* television show, I naturally jumped at the chance. It was a wonderful opportunity to combine my love of both animals and the beautiful Scottish Highlands. I started work on the show just before the first lockdown in March 2020 and like everyone, I had to adapt to changing times fast. With the help of my husband Kevin, I was able to set up a studio at home, and the *Highland Vet* recording sessions aided by my 'soundman' became a bright spot in what was otherwise a rather gloomy time.

The dedication of Guy and his team was inspiring to see. Working in all weathers across thousands of miles from the most northerly mainland veterinary practice in the UK, the stories of puppies, seals and the like being restored to health were heart-warming and uplifting. Like many people who have seen the show, I feel as if I know the Thurso vets very well. I recognise and admire their passion, skill and commitment to their work. The show was honoured with a Royal Television Society Award in 2021, which proves that many others too have fallen in love with this gem of a series.

Further fascinating insights to what the life of a Highland vet involves can be gleaned from the following pages, which reveal the challenges that these exceptional people face from day to day, working with the animals of the homes, farms and wild areas of northern Scotland. It has been my joy and honour to be involved with *The Highland Vet*, and I very much hope you will enjoy reading the book.

Phyllis Logan

Chapter One

In and Out of Shadow

It's Monday morning in D. S. McGregor & Partners' Thurso surgery and I'm preparing for an unusually demanding day ahead. Vet Rebecca is assessing the four animals that spent the night and will then put on her scrubs to join me in the operating room. Elsewhere, vet Fiona is wrestling with a full diary of routine appointments in our consulting area, and vet Ken is on his way to the local Veterinary Investigation Laboratory, where several post-mortem examinations await him. Out on large-animal calls, vet William is adding to his considerable career tally of horn and testicle removals, and vets Bridget, Pietro, Eilidh and David are about to spread themselves right across the farms and fields of Caithness and north Sutherland, assuming the varying roles of surgeon, podiatrist, dentist, medic or midwife as each situation dictates.

It's a typically manic start to the week in our Scottish Highlands practice.

Luckily, we haven't had any emergencies to squeeze into our already full 9am time slot, but the walk-ins and 'I need an answer now' type phone calls have been simply relentless, tying up all our receptionists' time and trickling down a constant feed of questions and concerns to today's in-house vets.

'Gregor from last week says his dog is still limping, Rebecca.'

'Fiona, Marjory wants to know if Tiddles the rabbit had a good night last night.'

'Guy, the man from yesterday is back with his greyhound again, says she's still not right. Any chance you can take a look?'

It's all a far cry from the practice I joined in the late 1990s. Back then, about this time of day, one of the senior partners, a stalwart of the profession, would be brusquely instructing us with words to the effect of 'Get surgery wrapped up by midday and get out on the farms to do some proper vetting.'

These days we can scarcely make our way through the long list of routine pet appointments without fielding a thousand other ancillary pet questions, let alone think about completing the surgical list before lunch and freeing up all the vets for work in the often all-too-fresh Caithness air.

The truth is, the animal-keeping habits of people have changed profoundly in the 24 years since I first started work up here in Thurso. There are quite simply a lot more pets, and pet owners today are a lot more clued-up as to what vets can do for them. As a result, people are much more willing to go the extra mile for the health and well-being of the animal they care for, and, for so many more people today, their pets are on equal footing with the human members of their family.

We, too, strive to provide the best care for the treasured companions presented to us, and so these manic mornings are here to stay. We accept the interruptions and the tasks shoehorned into our schedules as part of working life; but if there's one time when staff know they should find someone else to answer their queries, it's probably when I'm deeply engrossed inside someone's pet with my surgical tools.

Today will not be a typical day for me, though. Shortly I'll be performing a surgical procedure that will be very long, complicated and intense. This is the type of challenge that sustains my passion for the job, but nonetheless, I'll admit that my adrenaline level is already higher than average. I can only hope it serves to increase my focus.

If there even is such a thing as a 'comfort zone' for a veterinary surgeon, then for me, this particular operation definitely lies somewhere on the extreme edge of it.

Our county, Caithness, forms the very peak of the great flat cap that sits on top of the head of Scotland, and Thurso is its northernmost town, which makes us the northernmost vets in all of mainland Britain.

Thurso is the end of the road (well, the end of the A9 at least) and faces out to sea from one extreme of our Great British land mass. Beyond us lie the Orkney Islands, and if you maintain that north-easterly line you will encounter the Shetland Islands too. Continue further still and you'll enter a vast tract of desolate Norwegian Sea, which won't see you strike landfall until you eventually meet the Svalbard archipelago, its polar bears, and the great snow and ice of the Arctic Circle.

Staring north from our shore pulls your gaze into a rare space: an unfathomably large area of oceanic wilderness where whalers once battled, Norsemen once roamed, and where open sea eventually met ice fields that were once presumed endless.

The idea of what really constitutes the 'extreme' north, or the truly remote, is all relative, of course. The modern world has played its role in bringing everyone just that little bit closer together, especially since the advent of the internet, with its social media, video calling, and online shopping.

To a Shetlander, we Caithness folk have doubtless always been seen as 'southerners', living out a relatively metropolitan and well-connected existence, but for people down in England, perhaps they may still view a visit to Edinburgh or Glasgow as them arriving in the proper 'north'.

We've actually had friends visiting Edinburgh suggest they 'pop up' to see us. We've then had to point out that would actually involve a journey of over 250 miles further north! For those that don't live here, it can often be a surprise to discover that Scotland stretches long on its journey towards the roof of the earth. I imagine it's a fact that dawns fairly heavily on those hardy souls who attempt to walk or cycle the entire length of Britain, especially when they cross the Scottish border and discover they are scarcely over halfway through their challenge.

Before my family moved up here, I can very well remember worrying that Thurso might have been a bridge too far. It was a significant step away from what I'd formerly perceived to be real 'civilisation' back in my previous jobs in central Scotland; but, as I now enjoy my third decade up here, it is much clearer to me that the true essence of what civilisation should aspire to be is encapsulated in a community such as this.

I initially found the advert for this job listed in the back pages of the British Veterinary Association's journal, the *Veterinary Record*. There was no location specified, just a box number to post your application to and a few very general words describing a position within a 'mixed practice in Scotland'. I applied and can well remember laughing when I discovered the job was actually at the very top of the country.

My wife, Jennifer, is from the Highlands, so we were hardly complete newcomers to the far north and its often unique isolation. However, at that point in my life, the furthest I had actually been upcountry was Helmsdale, which we visited on our honeymoon. I hadn't even set foot in the county of Caithness, let alone made it as far Thurso; but if you simply looked on a map, you'd be forgiven for thinking the leap from Helmsdale to Thurso was hardly a big deal.

Superficially, at least, they were both pretty far up Scotland already, and sat just 40 miles apart. Down on the ground, though, you soon realised why those 40 miles felt like *such* a wild leap beyond.

The Causeway Mire, or 'Cazziemire' as it is pronounced by the locals, is a giant blackened mass of marsh, peatland and bog that effectively severs Thurso from the rest of the world. On my first car journey across the Causeway Mire, I felt like I had been cast adrift on a vast, lonely ocean.

It's a landscape more befitting of some wild, windswept Arctic tundra, not Scotland, and just a couple of miles of driving within this eerily bleak expanse made me wonder whether I was making a very big mistake indeed.

Where on *earth* was I going? Could I really work all the way out *here*? What about my family? What about our children? How were they going to get on in this seemingly brutal wilderness? It felt completely crazy to even be going for an interview, let alone actually be considering *taking a job.*

As I broke the back of the county, and the Causeway Mire, the landscape gradually evolved into gently rolling farmland. Soon, I could sense the coastline ahead, and then Thurso appeared on the horizon.

It was like spying a lighthouse, or a snug-looking harbour, just as you thought your drifting vessel would never see land-fall again. Instantly, I felt enormously reassured. People really did live up here, and, as I would later find out, they were very friendly people indeed.

Up here, we may be isolated, but we are never lonely. The nature of where we live means people really do look out for one another. They do take care and 'check in'. There is a genuine sense of commonality and unity at the core of what makes our commu-nity tick. When we first arrived, there was very much a sense that the community was self-sufficient, and, to an extent, that can still be said, although internet shopping has significantly changed that – and will continue to do so, no doubt.

We have everything that's actually necessary to enjoy life (who really needs two dozen different types of the same breakfast cereal anyway?) and, quite honestly, we've always been able to find nearly everything we want just in Thurso and Caithness. If we do ever need a taste of the big city, then Inverness is hardly on the moon. In fact, my mother-in-law, living within half an hour of Inverness, has on occasion *chosen* to do her Christmas shopping up here instead!

The funny thing about adjusting to a place that once seemed completely isolated is that you either can't cope and thus leave, or it eventually begins to feel like home, and the edges it once had just slip away.

It was the end of 1997 when I took the job in Thurso and our life changed. On discussing newcomers to the area, my colleagues frequently comment that people who move here must be prepared to give it time, and, above all, that they must give it at least a couple of winters. Such was the case with my family. I liked the place of course, but I didn't fall in love with Thurso and Caithness instantly; rather, over the period of a few years, our roots deepened into the earth here, until one day I came to the realisation that I really couldn't ever imagine leaving.

It was a pattern we shared with many people who moved here from other parts – most notably the 'atomics', workers who were first brought here to fill positions at the newly constructed Dounreay nuclear power station back in the mid-1950s. Originally, the organisation in charge of constructing the sites felt the need to offer financial incentives to motivate people to take a job at such a far-flung location. Now, as we welcome a fourth generation of those atomic descendants, and the Dounreay plant continues with a long phase of decommissioning, it's abundantly clear that no such encouragement was ever needed to make people stay.

It isn't for everyone, though, and the harsh winters soon sort out those who came here with romantic images of living out some 'good life' fantasy, with a smallholding, chickens and home-baked bread. It is different, but that difference quite often is what makes life up here so very special.

One of my earliest memories of quite how different things could be in Thurso was when I went into the bank and requested an overdraft so we might be able to buy a house. We couldn't have been living here for more than a couple of months, certainly not long enough, in my mind, for people to know who we were and certainly not long enough for the extreme act of faith that was coming.

We fully expected to be asked to return for an appointment, to show some formal identification, a work contract or, at the very least, evidence that we had the means to pay back a debt. However, as I began to make my request to the cashier, a woman from behind a different desk simply shouted over, 'Yeah, that's fine. How much do you want?'

We hadn't even given our names!

Somewhat taken aback, I stammered a figure in reply, which was cheerfully accepted and then she walked off entirely. Jennifer and I didn't really know what to do, so we just left too. Feeling pretty confused about the whole exchange, we resolved to just try again another day.

A few days later a letter hit our doormat confirming our overdraft was all in place. The jungle drums had clearly been beating behind the scenes, and everyone must have been quite aware that I was the new local vet, but even now it feels pretty extraordinary that they knew enough about us on sight alone to dispense with all the formalities. That's the way it is up here, though, and is illustrative of how warm and hospitable a small Highland community can really be.

Thurso is no yokel's backwater, but it does have an outpost feel. Much of the town is built on a grid system, not dissimilar to the style of many American towns and cities, and the veterinary surgery sits on land just off one of the grid's corners, over on the west bank of Thurso's river and between the secondary school, the railway station and the bus depot.

Ours is a practical building. Housed beneath metal profile roofing, we have a reception area, waiting room, consulting rooms, prep room, kennels and operating room. Connected to these by a corridor is our large-animal wing, which we refer to as 'the lambing shed', whatever the season, as this is a major activity that occurs there. Here we care for animals taken in from over 1,000 square miles of farms, smallholdings, moorland, villages and the town of Thurso itself. To describe the practice simply as 'mixed' is probably playing down the extraordinary breadth of cases we see through our doors and on our rounds. It can be anything from the traditional (sheep, horses and cows; pet cats and dogs), to the exotic and unusual (snakes, lizards, turtles and tortoises), to the wild (raptors with broken wings, deer hit by cars, and, in the wintertime, disorientated and malnourished seal pups).

The list of species and breeds the vets here might end up treating through the course of their career could run well over a hundred, and the number of individuals will run into the tens of thousands, but there will always be those special few cases that you can never forget.

Like the one that was limping across our car park today.

Shadow is a four-year-old Belgian Shepherd, looked after by his very concerned-looking owner, Andrew. He explained that Shadow had damaged a joint on his hind leg when he'd recently leapt into a river.

It was his hock joint, and the chief reason for my concern about this operation was the sheer complexity of this area. Many little bones, each forming a joint with its neighbour, make up the hock.

Study a dog's rear leg and you'll notice it fairly obviously: travel down from the dog's hip and find its knee joint (the stifle) and then, further down still, you'll locate an angular, backwards-pointing articulation – that's the hock. It could be mistaken for some kind of rear elbow by those who haven't studied anatomy, but it is actually the equivalent of our ankle, with its point matching our heel.

What you have to understand is that dogs are actually standing as a human would if we were permanently walking on our toes. It means all of those intricate toe bone structures that we have on the flats of our feet are travelling from the paw, up the dog's leg and on into the hock. Incidentally, horses and cows go one stage further and actually walk as a ballerina, *en pointe*.

Accessing the many joints, and gaining purchase on the many small bones with the implants required for a repair, is a real challenge from a surgical point of view. What mattered to me most with Shadow was achieving that access and managing to securely fix metalwork that would withstand his use of the leg while it all healed.

The surgery Shadow required is known as arthrodesis. It was evident from the physical examination and X-rays that he had a dislocation within his hock and the damage was far beyond the body's ability to repair itself with simple treatment. The only way forward was to effectively fuse the joint. I would need to stabilise the region with a steel plate, and then ask his body to heal two formerly jointed bones into one single longer bone. Such inter-tarsal joints are low-motion at the best of times and so fusing this one would barely affect Shadow's movement in the long term; it was a joint he could afford to lose, and currently he was struggling to bear any weight on that leg at all.

I had conducted many less complex arthrodesis operations before, but Shadow's hock was a step up. His separation had occurred between the bones known as the proximal tarsals. If the damage had been any more extensive then it really wouldn't have been up for discussion at all. I would've been forced to turn Andrew and Shadow away, and they'd have needed to go elsewhere to find a specialist surgeon.

The issue up here, though, is what 'elsewhere' really means for a pet owner. We are not just the most northerly vet practice on the mainland; we probably have a fairly good shot at being among the most isolated. The only other surgery close to us is our sister practice over in Wick. Although having two branches might mean that animal owners can usually get to us within half an hour of anywhere within Caithness, pursuing specialist treatment further afield not only can be a logistical challenge but also could take time a sick animal might not have, and is potentially a lot more expensive too.

This is not something we ever take lightly. If the buck truly stops with us, then we make sure we are always giving the highest standards of care possible. There are limitations: no one here would take on a procedure they didn't have at least some confidence in or elementary experience of; but it means that we have to accept that, in cases like Shadow's, there may be times we have to do things that vets in better-connected parts of the nation would be much more likely to pass up the chain to a specialist.

A few years ago, I was faced with the prospect of conducting a thoracotomy on a dog: a surgical procedure where I had to open up the animal's chest and operate within an inch of the heart. It was definitely a job which, had we been almost anywhere else in mainland Scotland, would've gone straight into the hands of a specialist.

The owner had recently moved to Thurso, was settling into a new job, and didn't have a huge amount of money, or time, when his dog accidentally swallowed a large fish hook. By the time this hook had caught hold within the dog, it was stuck firm within his oesophagus, halfway down his chest.

We tried everything to get this fish hook to shift naturally, but because it was barbed it just wasn't going to happen. We looked at sending the dog to a vet on Orkney to attempt to get it out via the throat with an endoscope, but they cautioned that, due to the barb on the point of the hook, you could easily end up tearing the oesophagus wide open on retrieval. I cast my net further afield, speaking to referral centres in Inverness, but no one there seemed to have an adequate answer either. One thing was for sure, though: to do nothing would have almost certainly led to a dangerous infection, which would likely have spread from the oesophagus into the chest cavity, ultimately resulting in the death of the dog.

It was one of those 'Right, let's just get on with it then' moments. There was absolutely no point worrying about it or taking any more time to deliberate. We were out of all other options, and I steeled myself to undertake what I'm fairly sure was the first thoracotomy ever conducted by a vet in Caithness.

It's not super-technical surgery in terms of the fine skills required, but there was no getting away from the fact it was going to mean opening up the dog's chest and heading into an entirely unfamiliar area – from my surgical perspective, at least. We knew the dog's lungs would collapse as soon as I entered his chest, so a nurse had to inflate and deflate them on his behalf – essentially, to 'breathe for him' throughout the surgery – and I had to try and synchronise all my actions to the rhythm of the lungs' movements.

As I timed my manoeuvres, the dog's heart was beating, right there, in front of my face, making me acutely aware that, in spite of the dramatic opening in the dog's chest, it was still very much alive, and that its aorta, the main artery leaving the heart, was directly next to the pipe that I was about to cut open in search of the hook.

I felt the precise location of the hook with my fingertips and managed to make a neat incision in the oesophagus. Removing it was only half the job. Next came the stitching, which needed to be undertaken with extreme care, to avoid heightening the risk of the oesophagus leaking through the wound, and to prevent it from ultimately healing with a 'stricture' – a scar that narrows its girth. There was a sense of both relief and achievement when the brave move paid off and the dog went on to make a full recovery.

As rare and as nerve-racking as moments like that undoubt-edly are, they do give a deep sense of job satisfaction when you get an animal successfully back on its feet against the odds. It is definitely something worth remembering when those challenges come around again, like they had today, with Shadow.

Before a procedure all we can really do is present the full and honest facts to the animal owners and then allow them to make their own decision over what they want to do – what is known as 'informed consent'. When it came to Shadow, Andrew didn't miss a beat.

'No need for a specialist, Guy,' he said, confidently penning his signature and handing me back the procedural consent forms. 'I trust you. I've seen you on the TV!'

We both laughed (me slightly more nervously than Andrew).

I took Shadow by his lead and persuaded him into the surgery building. Michelle, one of our nursing assistants, helped keep him calm while I conducted all the basic observations: weighing him, checking him over physically, listening to his chest. Then I took a pre-anaesthetic blood sample to screen for any hidden abnormalities in his blood, liver or kidneys. All of this is standard pre-operative procedure. It helps us determine whether an animal's body really is in good enough shape to handle a long operation and the duration of anaesthetic it requires.

With that successfully completed, I could then administer a 'pre-med' to Shadow, which included a pain reliever (to help manage his discomfort during the procedure) and a sedative (to help calm him down, for both his sake and ours).

It's really important that any animal is as relaxed as possible at the start of any operation as, firstly, we wish to reduce its anxiety and, secondly, we generally need to administer an anaesthetic using an intravenous (IV) cannula, which would be troublesome to feed into a vein in a panicked and jumpy patient.

Twenty minutes after I've administered the pre-med, Shadow is lying on the operating room table in a state of total calm. Gently, I cannulate him, feeding the small plastic tube into a vein on his front leg. His tongue rolls out of his mouth and he stares happily into the middle distance. Then, from a large syringe, I begin to allow the anaesthetic to flow into his system. 'There you go, fella,' I whisper calmly, 'the magic juice to make you go to sleep.'

If it were a very quick procedure, like nipping the wart off a dog's body, that IV anaesthetic alone would be enough to keep a patient under for the entire operation, but the hours needed to perform the complex surgery on Shadow's hock require what we call a 'maintenance phase' of anaesthesia.

As soon as Shadow falls asleep, we quickly intubate him by inserting a tube into his windpipe, effectively keeping his airway open and giving us total control over what he inhales. Through that tube we can then maintain Shadow's life, and state of peaceful ignorance to the procedure, by administering him a mix of oxygen and anaesthetic gas. This maintenance phase will ensure he remains comfortably unconscious for the entire duration of the operation, and that the continued delivery of that anaesthetic, plus the monitoring of his heart and breathing rate, can now be left to one of our attentive and qualified nurses.

With Shadow finally fully under, I take a moment to look at his hock once more. 'Well, there you go,' I say out loud, as I gently manipulate the joint. 'We have a bend in a place where there shouldn't be a bend.'

The nurses prepare Shadow, cutting back the hair around his hock with clippers and then sterilising the operating area by scrubbing it with a surgical-grade disinfectant. The operation itself may take several hours, and just getting an animal fully ready for a procedure can in itself take 45 additional minutes. It's a long time, but, once I'm in the zone, time really does fly. In fact, as my focus intensifies, I'll often lose track of time altogether, though the nurses will always keep me aware of how long we've been going.

I pick up my scalpel and make my first cut along the skin over Shadow's hock. A small rivulet of crimson-red blood spills down his fur-free and sterilised skin, and, as I deepen the opening, the true extent of the problem I foresaw during my external observations is revealed.

Shadow has grown a thick lump beneath his skin that extends right across the damaged portion of his hock. It is a dense, grisly thickening in the ligament that normally supports this region and was his body's natural response to compensate for the collapse. However, it presents a bit of a surgical nightmare. Negotiating normal ligaments to access this joint is tough enough, but getting past this rigid lump is going to be like teasing through the fibres of an old ship's rope.

I reach for my periosteal elevator: a small hand tool that looks a little like a small metal spatula with a slightly curved head and an exceptionally sharp edge. Ostensibly, it's designed to lift the periosteum, a dense supportive layer of tissue that covers bones, but it is equally useful here.

Steel meets tissue and I begin the task of lifting away ligament from Shadow's ankle bones.

Chapter Two

Grafting to the Bone

I mine deeper into Shadow's hock and his blood flows readily and steadily. I wipe it away regularly with a gauze swab so it doesn't pool in the open wound and obscure my view.

With Shadow, we have an anaesthesia nurse monitoring the dog and his gas, a theatre nurse preparing and handing me all the tools for the job, a second operating vet supporting me surgically, and then me, the veterinary surgeon, conducting the operation itself. Everyone needs to understand the procedure and the importance of their own role in giving the operation the very best chance of success. The best nurses and surgical assistants are the ones that have such a keen sense of the procedure and its demands that they can almost read my mind.

Fleece-white surgical swabs quickly turn a deep red and onwards I dissect, shredding through fibrous ligament and getting ever closer to those separated bones.

Controlling your natural instincts at the sight of a lot of blood is something which only really comes with time and training, but it always pays to be vigilant, even when you're operating well within your skill level and experience.

Just this week, I was coaching a new young vet in how to spay a bitch, a routine procedure that involves removing the uterus and ovaries from a female dog. Sure enough, there I was overseeing her perform this entry-level, yet unnervingly tricky, operation, when suddenly, one of the clamps on a major blood vessel popped clean off. The freshly liberated artery pinged back into the animal's abdomen, as if it were an elastic band flicked across a classroom by a naughty schoolkid.

Blood really can pump like a hose in such situations, but, with a new graduate right in front of me, it was imperative that I maintained my cool.

'Ah, these things happen,' I said, with what I hoped was a breezy tone, and then off we went fishing for the free-squirting blood vessel secreted somewhere inside the dog.

Of course, we quickly caught and clamped the little blighter and the procedure was completed with absolutely no ill effect to the dog. Ultimately, it was just one of those things you must learn to handle; even with the greatest plans and set-ups, unexpected things will very occasionally still occur.

With all the thick ligament moved away to provide access, I can finally get down to the job of removing Shadow's articular cartilage: the flexible shock-absorbing tissue coating the inner surface of his dislocated ankle joint. Vet Rebecca, my second, cranks open the joint and allows me to go ever deeper with my tools: a diamond-tipped drill, a sharp-edged Volkmann's scoop, a pair of precision tweezers and the trusty periosteal elevator.

Soon, the blunt sound of metal scraping bone, like a climber grinding their sharp pickaxe against rock, fills the operating room. We're getting there, but operations like this always feel like there's an awful lot of destruction before any actual fixing of the issue can begin in earnest.

Shadow remains utterly compliant and blissfully unconscious. His breathing is stable, and his great tongue is still flopped out on my operating table, remaining a reassuring shade of pink.

It can feel counter-intuitive as a surgeon, especially one who is usually so meticulous in their efforts to not cause any damage to an animal, when you're tearing off healthy cartilage and deliberately ruining joint surfaces, but this, I know, all must be done. It would be a futile attempt at an arthrodesis if I were to leave the cartilage intact; any remaining cartilage would act as a permanent barrier to the bones ever fusing together and healing as one.

Even with something as well known as a hip replacement, you're still having to chop off the gammy hip before you can replace it with a prosthesis. These are 'salvage procedures', not operations intending to work with, or encourage the healing of, an original joint, bone or organ. All salvage procedures involve a certain element of destruction before the restoration and repair can actually begin.

It takes a certain type of personality to make peace with that difficult reality. It is definitely not an obvious aspect of the profession when a young, hopeful teenager first makes the decision to pursue veterinary surgery as a career.

I have been fascinated by animals for as long as I can remember – not just farm animals or pets but literally every kind of animal I could possibly engage with in the environment that was around me. It didn't matter if they were the animals in our home, in my garden, or on the television; I was captivated by them all.

I was born in the English military town of Aldershot. My mum and dad had met while working in the army, as a nurse and a radiographer respectively, but when I turned four, they began their civilian careers. We went briefly to Edinburgh, then Doncaster, before eventually settling in Lancashire, but no matter where we went, I always took that love of animals with me.

My dream growing up was to be the next Sir David Attenborough, but as I started to progress through school, my enjoyment of all the science subjects, coupled with this passion for animals, led people around me to say, 'Oh, Guy, you'll be a vet when you grow up.' It's funny how often comments can stick with a child deep into their adulthood.

During school I took on work experience at my local veterinary practice. It certainly didn't put me off; in fact, my interest in becoming a vet grew markedly. However, before going on to study veterinary medicine at the University of Edinburgh, I was fortunate enough to take a rare opportunity to work abroad in Eswatini, the southern African kingdom then known as Swaziland, and gained some first-hand experience with many of the iconic big-game animals.

There were moments in my life when I did consider going down a more purely scientific route or, perhaps better still, becoming a zoo vet. Both seemed exciting and exotic, but honestly, I have absolutely no regrets at how it has all worked out.

Age and experience have taught me to be careful what you wish for. The grass is not always greener on the other side and no one really has it all. Even Sir David Attenborough, with his perfect broadcasting career, has in recent years spoken of his sadness at missing his children grow up. Working in Thurso has taught me the enormous benefits of having one place to really call home, and I can also see now that choosing to pursue this career path might, quite counter-intuitively, have thrown up just as many extraordinary moments as I would have encountered in a zoo.

I married before my final year at university, and children arrived during my early years as a qualified vet. The demands of a domestic practice, with its long hours and nights on call, kept me out of my home more than I would have liked. However, the Attenborough lifestyle, and even potentially that of a specialist zoo vet, may have limited family life even more.

In domestic mixed practice, I've revelled in the challenges thrown at me, I've enjoyed feeling part of a community and I've had immense job satisfaction treating and repairing the more familiar species. I've also been able to be a dad and a husband. You really can't ask for much more than that.

Shadow is going to need a bone graft to help aid the arthrodesis. Carefully, I incise the skin and expose the bone at the top of Shadow's tibia on his good leg, then drill a small hole to allow me to scoop out the spongy material sequestered deep under the hard surface.

It isn't necessary to collect a huge amount; just a few small gooey samples will be enough. I may be continuing the theme of doing damage for the greater long-term good, yet the soreness he's likely to experience from this small procedure will be surprisingly minimal.

With Shadow's tibia bone material successfully extracted, I mix it in a small pot together with his blood and some powdered bone I pre-ordered from a tissue bank, a storage facility for pet tissue from deceased donor animals. This putty-like mixture will supercharge the healing process and massively increase Shadow's chances of a successful bone fusion. Carefully, I spread the semi-solid pink blend into Shadow's defaced joint space, before asking the theatre nurse for my drill, some screws and a steel plate ordered specifically for this job.

Finally, I can make the floppy joint before me entirely rigid.

'Guy,' a voice, distinct from any of the veterinary staff, whispers out from the corner of the room. 'Can you tell me what's going on, please?' The voice comes from somewhere behind a high-definition camera and belongs to the self-shooting director in charge of filming the operation today.

I can clearly remember the afternoon, a couple of years ago now, when Lynda the receptionist placed a hand over the surgery phone's receiver and excitedly whispered, 'Guy! It's the people who make *The Yorkshire Vet*. They want to speak to you!'

It was Daisybeck Studios, the Leeds-based production company responsible for the extremely popular Channel 5 series *The Yorkshire Vet*, and it now appeared that they wanted to spread their wings further north.

Looking back, our out-of-the-way location, the unique mix of animals and all the local characters made a persuasive case for filming at our surgery, but at the time, I'll admit I had mixed feelings about the prospect of inviting cameras up here.

Being on television wasn't something that had ever occurred to any of us. It certainly wasn't a dream of mine, and, if I'm honest, I worried about the crew getting in the way of our work and how I might feel if they ended up making us all look a bit daft by over-dramatising what we did.

I think I was fairly cool about it all on the phone to Daisybeck. They sent on a questionnaire for me to fill in about our practice and work, but I only managed to fill out half before I went on holiday with Jennifer.

I was pretty certain the whole thing was just going to blow over into nothing and that we'd never hear from them again. However, when I returned from holiday, I discovered my half-hearted attempt at their lengthy questionnaire had obviously not dissuaded them; they'd even been up and filmed some taster sequences with Ken, the other company director in Thurso alongside myself.

They now wanted to come back to film with me, and that really was the moment I knew I'd just have to take a leap of faith.

Within reason, I always think you should try to take every opportunity that comes your way in life. It may flop or turn out not to be worth continuing, but don't knock it back from the outset. You don't want to be remembered as the person who didn't join the Beatles or turned down J. K. Rowling, and I couldn't really turn this whole thing down purely on the basis of what I thought it might be like. I certainly wasn't going to find out if I didn't give it a chance. Besides, several of the staff were now very excited about the whole prospect. I took the plunge and we never really looked back.

Now, three Channel 5 seasons down the road, I have to say we have warmly welcomed Daisybeck and their crew into our working lives. They are genuinely nice people and lots of fun to have around. We are all really pleased with how brilliantly well the series is produced and put together, and I'm proud at the part it has played in educating the wider public about the everyday work we vets undertake.

More than anything, it's great to get this oft-overlooked corner of Scotland, its animals and its special community into people's homes. I have no regrets at all, but filming does add an extra dimension of pressure when we're working on the trickiest of our customers and have a camera whirring away in the corner.

It took a bit of getting used to, learning how to tailor my responses to not make them too long or technical, and how to phrase an answer without it seeming like I've just been asked a question by the director. It probably took an adjustment for the camera crew, too, both looking through the lens at an often gory scene and coming to terms with the fact that there are times that we just can't answer their questions due to the immediacy of the medical problem we're dealing with.

No matter what, we all agreed that caring for the animals *must* come first, and we were determined that production of *The Highland Vet* would not slow down any essential procedure, especially one live on the operating table.

At this point in Shadow's operation, I can take a breath. I'm between the two main stages – destruction and stabilisation – so it's safe to say a few words to the camera about what's going on and how we're all doing.

If anything, when it comes to operations as long and complex as Shadow's, I actually get the sense the camera crew might get a little bored sometimes. Certainly, as the minutes become hours, one crew member might slink off for lunch, but at least one cameraperson will always remain to catch the critical stages of any operation, and, with Shadow's leg now ready to take the plate and screws, we have just reached one of those moments.

I position the plate across the joint. It was manufactured flat and so needs to be contoured (bent, in other words) to fit the profile of the bones' surface. I use large lever-like plate benders to repeatedly tweak the plate then try it against the bone until I'm happy with the fit.

The plate is long and rectangular but tapered at the end where it will sit over the narrower toe bones, and it has eight neat holes for the screws. Superficially, it looks like the most extortionately priced piece of children's Meccano, but this little plate will help make sure Shadow's bones fuse in-line, just as soon as I've screwed it down.

'Let's get one screw in place,' I call across to Rebecca. 'The critical one is the central one. Get that in a good place and everything else will follow.'

This is no mean feat. On the surface it might look like I'm simply using the plate to bridge the gap between two obvious bones, but deeper into the hock joint are other small bones, and this central screw ideally needs to penetrate the first bone and then grip a second, which is both out of view and minuscule.

I look to Shadow's original X-rays and make a series of minute adjustments to the position of the plate. The margin for error here is practically zero, and any inaccuracy might seriously diminish Shadow's chances of a full recovery, but I remind myself that the most important thing is that I achieve a firm purchase with this first screw.

Rebecca supports the hock joint and holds the plate in its final position while I reach for the drill.

One more bit of real focused effort now, and we're well on the home straight.

As I head into what I suppose I have to reluctantly admit is the more senior end of my career, I have found myself reflecting a lot more on what it takes to be a vet.

I think being armed with an intensely curious yet methodical mind is one really useful trait. I've always been fired up by the diagnostic, Sherlock Holmes side of vetting, where you are trying to find the culprit, search for what's wrong, identify the cause of the malady and then, hopefully, fix it successfully.

Having a passion for animals is a really obvious thing too, but there is a massive caveat here that a lot of people don't consider: you will be quickly broken if you can't find at least some way to maintain an emotional distance from the animal you're working with.

Unfortunately, we do see some desperately sad cases, just as you would in the human medical world. Sometimes we see animals in a terrific amount of pain as well, and often, as with Shadow, further discomfort after a visit to the practice is inevitable, though we do our best to control it medically.

Just because animals don't always express emotions in the same way we do doesn't mean that they don't experience emotion. You will witness animals with very real feelings of terror, confusion and deep uncertainty and anxiety.

Remember, too, that barring the wildlife we treat, every animal also comes with an owner, and, for many pet owners, the loss of that animal can be equivalent to losing a dearly loved family member. Being sympathetic and empathetic to their grief, while keeping your own professional objectivity, is not something that comes naturally to everyone, especially if you entered this profession because you thought you were only going to 'work with animals'.

None of that means a good vet is one who is cold or lacking in compassion. I still find it hard when I see an animal suffering, and I've spent many sleepless nights pondering the most challenging of my cases. I'm human too, and I can remember so many times when I've been with a truly heartbroken owner as they've said goodbye to a beloved pet; but as difficult as any loss is to take, as a vet there are always many other sick animals waiting for your full attention and care. You simply *must* find ways to cope and move on if you are to continue to be of service to the next, and then the next, animal and its owner.

Some people just can't do it, and there is no shame in that. I see it in one of my own daughters. Like me, she absolutely adores animals, but she openly admits she could never handle seeing an animal in any pain. Even as a young adult, there are still certain films that she will point-blank refuse to watch because she has been forewarned that an animal will die in them. She is far from alone in feeling this way – I guess millions of people do; in fact, I recently discovered that my brother has been fast-forwarding through episodes of *The Highland Vet*, just to see me in it, while avoiding any of the very occasional storylines where an animal didn't make it.

To those people who have that intensity of feeling and still want to become a vet, I have to warn you that you will need to develop a good dose of pragmatism, realism, and emotional resilience.

You can and will do your absolute best, but some animals will die regardless of all your efforts, and dealing with that, I'm afraid to say, is very much part of what it takes to be a vet.

The other side, though, is the extraordinary and inimitable buzz you feel when you do manage to turn it all around for an animal in your care. It isn't just a sterile feeling of scientific accomplishment when you save a life; you feel a real intense and palpable joy, especially when you later see how the animal is thriving and how happy your work has made its owner.

That pleasure is a natural human reaction you thankfully don't have to suppress, and is a huge reason why we all do this job. Those memories of all the good outcomes can really help carry you through the darker times.

I wash my hands in the prep-room basin and breathe a huge sigh of relief that Shadow's operation is finally over.

The seven remaining screws have been placed successfully and the metal plate has rigidly bridged the gap across Shadow's joint. It feels very solid and stable now, a real contrast to the hock of the poor animal that hobbled into the surgery first thing this morning.

I glance up at the clock. Another missed lunch. Should I just have a quick cup of tea, keep going, and wait until dinner to refuel myself?

The operation took over three hours from the first cut to the last stitch, but 'time' as a vet often fits within its own special little conceptual realm. On the one hand, the time it just took to conduct Shadow's surgery whistled past, but on the other, the intensity of focus it required often felt so great, it was almost as if the clock could have stopped entirely. It was seriously gruelling at points (I certainly sweated a fair bit too) but the time has now come to take a break, crack a joke and loosen up after the tension of such a long period of high concentration.

Mug in hand, I ponder how intense our work can be at times. Springtime is our busy season, when new lambs and calves arrive in abundance. A cup of tea like this, let alone lunch, can feel like a real luxury.

Following the relentless spring rush, things don't really slow again until the summer, when the holidaymakers arrive with their pets and their own unique challenges. Then, before you know it, it's getting colder, wetter, and windier once more. The cattle are brought under cover, the wildlife calls are dominated by stranded seal pups, and the long, dark nights take hold of the Highlands again. Such is the circle of life for the Highland vet.

Time, in this veterinary practice, does tend to follow something of a seasonal pattern, but even so, after almost a quarter of a century working here, I've come to learn that you should never be a slave to the calendar or the clock. The lives and troubles of animals, as with their human custodians, are guided by that unpredictable and random element of chaos. Throw on top of that the indiscriminate climate of the far north, and the only thing you can really rely on is that no one week, season or year will ever be quite the same as the one before.

I dry my hands and glance again at our schedule for the remainder of the day. It looks manageable, but even a routine operation can suddenly grow arms and legs and become something much more complicated. There's really no way of knowing what will come through the door, or down the phone lines, next.

I wholly believe this must be one of the most rewarding professions, though, and for the people who choose to work in this type of veterinary practice in particular, the thrill of that great unknown is another one of the many things that keep us coming in day after day and year after year.

I take a sip of my tea and look out of the window. It's raining again, but no matter what comes our way, our work also takes place in one of the most captivating landscapes I've ever witnessed.

Even on the worst of days up here, it's very hard to feel anything but blessed.

Hogmanay

Chapter Three

A New Year

The Highlands of Scotland.

The name conjures up iconic images of enormous snow-capped mountains; wide, sloping pine-filled glens; and giant windswept lochs, all splitting the landscape in every direction you care to turn.

When you travel up through Scotland, it is possible to get a sense of an ever-increasing scale. Feast on the beauty of the Borders, the prettiness of Perthshire, then the cool-capped Cairngorms. Yet the perception of sheer, unrestrained vastness increases the further north you venture. Rugged peaks continue to adorn the north and the west, but if you then turn to the extreme north-east, and head into our corner of the land, it may seem that parts have been quite abruptly flattened by a heavy roller.

It was a revelation to realise this area, with less of a vertical vista to capture the eye, is very special in its own right. Mountains may be two a penny elsewhere in this nation, but there is only one Flow Country.

Covering most of Caithness and a portion of Sutherland, the Flow Country's enormous expanse of open wetlands constitutes the largest blanket bog in the whole of Europe. Named after the Old Norse word *floi*, meaning 'wet' or 'marshy', this area is critically important for biodiversity and plays a huge role in climate change mitigation, owing to its ability to capture carbon and lock it within beds of peat. In fact, it is estimated that these ancient peat bogs store around 400 million tonnes of carbon; that's more than double the amount stored in the whole of Britain's woodlands put together.

The sparsity of trees in this corner of Scotland will be noticed by incomers from the relatively well-forested south. The trees that are brave enough to grow here often do so with a permanent lean in the direction of the prevailing wind. The horizons are simply huge. With few trees, mountains or settlements to break the horizon, standing in the heart of the Flow Country always gives you an impressive feeling of wild open space, especially if you choose to come here on a good day in the very pit of winter.

Some of our very best days in Caithness can occur bang in the middle of our coldest season. Cold but windless, sunny, crisp and clear days are the absolute ideal. The marshy surface layers of the Flow Country freeze, and its grasses, marshes and pools become ossified atop the 10,000-year-old peat. Even on our portion of tidal river in Thurso, ice can form during persistent frosts, with chunks then breaking off and floating away as mini icebergs towards the estuary.

On the finest winter days you can see for many miles. In fact, the views are often clearer than those in the height of summer. With no haze coming off the sea, it's almost like you can feel the crags and lines that mark the cliff faces on the Orkney island of Hoy, some 15 miles from Thurso across the Pentland Firth. The sea can be as still and calm as a mill pond. So calm, in fact, that the Orkney Islands themselves really do feel just a few strong swimming strokes away. But the renowned danger of the Pentland currents and the shockingly cold salt water would conspire against such an excursion. I really wouldn't recommend it.

At other times, winter here can feel long, drawn out and wearisome. We have this classic Scottish word, 'dreich',* which sums up, really, in both its pronunciation and its meaning, the extreme gloominess of a bleak and often drizzly day. A day described as dreich doesn't have the punctuating drama of a gale or a snowstorm; it's more of an unremitting damp and dreary greyness.

No matter what the weather is doing, this high up the curve of the earth, you're certainly looking at a much shorter day in midwinter. In January, the morning light is only just breaking through when I'm starting work and is already failing again by mid-afternoon. If I'm working exclusively in the surgery during this time, then I'm unlikely to see much daylight at all.

If the shortest days meet with a long passage of dreich days, the distinction between day and night can really start to blur. Sometimes there is only a short period where it's simply 'less dark' and not really what you would call 'daylight' at all, just a dismal duskiness before the night falls properly. Those are the times that having plenty of personal and work-related preoccupations can really see you through.

Dreich. You can almost feel it percolate to your soul. If not that, then the often-punishing wind will drill into your core. Combine either with the short winter days and you understand the reason why people say that newcomers should spend at least a couple of winters in Caithness before committing to this place full-time.

---

* *Dreich*: Pronounced 'dreech', with a soft Scottish 'ch', as in 'loch'.

Thurso town understands how to endure a rough winter. It sits snugly in the corner of a C-shaped bay where a retreating tide reveals a golden sandy beach. A river cuts through its eastern edge, and the settlement dates right back to the Picts. In Viking times it would once have been a gateway to Scotland for the Norse folk. Indeed, historians generally acknowledge that 'Thurso' has its roots in the Viking word 'Thorsá', meaning 'river of the god Thor'. Thurso later evolved into a successful fishing town and an important trading hub, particularly famed for its Caithness flagstone: the Caithness 'slab', a Devonian sandstone which was exported to northern European ports right through to the nineteenth century. These iconic pieces of stone have an exceptional durability. For many generations long slabs were driven into the earth and used to form great stone walls to mark the boundaries between farmland, erupting from the earth like the great grey teeth of a giant. Many such walls are still standing today, but the high prices the stone soon commanded meant its local use was curtailed as the valuable trading markets expanded. Even today you can find Caithness flagstones in the Scottish Parliament, King's Cross station in London, and as far away as the streets of Sydney, Australia, and Boston Harbor in Massachusetts, USA.

Big changes came to Thurso in the 1950s with the opening of the nuclear power station at Dounreay. Situated 10 miles to the west, the plant and its influx of workers effectively trebled the population of the town, but nonetheless Thurso has always retained its cosiness and small-town feel. So many of Britain's urban expanses feel crowded, with no real sense of where one place begins and another one ends, but Thurso retains clearly defined boundaries, and its identity. Wick, 20 miles to the east, holds the title of county town, and is the only other town in a county scattered with villages and hamlets.

Thurso is a real place of comfort when the worst of the winter whips through the Highlands. Even now, I feel a sense of homely security when I see the lights of the town nestling cosily in the bay as I approach out of a long winter's darkness from a job deep in the countryside. It is the very same feeling I felt when I first laid eyes on the town, at the end of that long drive across the Causeway Mire all those years ago.

It is New Year's Day. Hogmanay, the Scots word for the last day of the old year, is over. Christmas trees are dropping their needles, wrapping paper fills our recycling bins, and here at the surgery we are starting to focus on the hope of a brighter new year.

It was a quieter Christmas than normal. The year had been notable worldwide for the coronavirus pandemic, and as we had made the big adjustments to mask wearing, social distancing and receiving our patients in the surgery car park, it's fair to say we were all anticipating that 2021 would see the nation really start to get on top of this awful virus.

It wasn't a lonely Christmas, though. Our, now grown-up, children had come to join us just before the latest wave of lockdowns really sank in over the Christmas period, with one of our girls even bringing her marooned university flatmate, from Indonesia, too. With the case rates really spiking by then, it looked as if they might end up hanging on in our home for rather longer than was originally planned. My wife and I felt really blessed. When the Christmas restrictions came into full force, the one day the government allowed people to meet up was on Christmas Day itself. A lot of people living in Thurso were not able to meet up with their families who live further afield, and we wouldn't have seen our girls at all if they hadn't decided to join us early.

It is very rare to see an animal late on Hogmanay itself. For that one night each year it really does have to be a dire emergency for an animal owner to call us out, but calls have occurred, or at least telephone advice given. So, if you are 'on call', a wee dram of whisky is not permitted! On New Year's Day mornings, people might often be too tired or hungover to realise that their animal would be best to see a vet before the holiday is over, but come the afternoon, calls can start to trickle in, and some of them can be really serious.

One New Year's Day I remember having to do an emergency hysterectomy on a cattle farmer's precious miniature poodle. The poor dog had an infection in her womb and required immediate surgery; pus was leaking into her abdominal cavity with potentially fatal consequences. It certainly required a steady hand and a clear head, and was a pertinent reminder that animals really don't follow the conventions and etiquettes laid down by the human calendar.

As January slides on this year, the festive period of the last few weeks soon starts to feel like a distant memory. We may be over the 'hump' of the shortest day, but the coldest months have really sunk their teeth into Caithness now, and this winter seems to be alternating between perishingly cold and just those really wet dreich days. These are the sorts of conditions where only the truly foolish would forsake their welly warmers, and, as a vet trained to use just one arm for cattle pregnancy diagnosis, you begin to wish you could warm up both your hands in the backside of a cow!

There are few greater metaphors for a fresh start, at the opening of a new year, than the birth of our first lambs. Even as early as January, the Caithness lambs will start to appear, and the first sheep breed to naturally produce those lambs is the Suffolk.

The Suffolk is a solid and stocky-looking sheep. It has a jet-black face, a tightly woven fine fleece, and a reputation for being a tough breed, capable of adapting to a whole host of conditions. Up here in Caithness, we only have a handful of Suffolk flocks when compared to the other commercial breeds we vets typically encounter later on in the spring.

According to the Suffolk Sheep Society, the breed itself has its origins right back in the late eighteenth century, when Suffolk farmers successfully crossed the Norfolk Horn ewe, one of the oldest sheep breeds in Britain, with the Southdown ram. In doing so, they created a cross that had excellent mutton, a far superior growth rate and an elemental hardiness that would later see the Suffolk sheep exported to nearly all the major sheep-rearing territories around the globe.

The ewe has a comparatively wide pelvis, which goes a long way to boosting any sheep's chances of having a natural and uncomplicated birth; but January does occasionally bring us some challenges with the Suffolks, particularly if there's a big single lamb on board. This year, I've been called to conduct a caesarean section on one poor ewe at three o'clock in the morning.

A caesarean section procedure is often abbreviated to 'C-section', but the vets and farmers up here simply know the operation as a 'Caesar'. Whether or not to conduct a Caesar on a sheep isn't always as straightforward a decision as you might think. There are plenty of grey areas where it remains in the balance whether to deliver naturally or to opt for surgery. However, there are also clear-cut cases where it is evidently impossible for a sheep to lamb naturally and there is little ambiguity over the likely outcome if a Caesar is not performed: it can be fatal for the lamb, and sometimes for the ewe too.

Often, we take the lead from the farmers who have brought in the sheep. Experienced lambers are very rarely wrong on these things, and given they are going to have to pay for the procedure, it isn't likely they'll take the decision to bring the sheep in on a whim. They will have already tried extracting the lamb through the rear portal, and you're a very brave vet if you opt to go against their wishes and attempt the same.

I'll tell you about all the ins and outs of the various awkward lamb positions and obstructions we can encounter once we are into the lambing season later this year, but suffice to say, the judgement that you make in those grey areas might be affected by things outwith the sphere of obstetrics. I once remember feeling inside a big Texel ewe who was experiencing birthing complications, when, as I was on the very cusp of making my decision whether or not to conduct the Caesar, the farmer leant in and gently reminded me that the twins inside her womb were likely to be worth £1,000. I'd like to think I wasn't swayed.

They were potentially prized male 'tup' lambs, and the price on the head (or rather, I should say, the testicles) of a high-quality breeding tup can be astronomic. To have on your farm a tup born from a long genetic line of proven breeders can make a great difference to the overall health and profitability of your entire flock, and farmers are willing to pay serious money for the privilege. In fact, just last summer a Texel tup at a Lanark auction was sold for an unprecedented 350,000 guineas. That's £367,500 in new money. (Livestock and racehorse auctions often quaintly retain the use of guineas, which were phased out of our routine currency over two centuries ago. Today a guinea is worth £1.05 and, I believe, the tradition is that the extra 5 per cent on the pound is the auctioneer's commission.)

In case you were wondering, with the aforementioned Texel, I opted for the Caesar.

Stephen, the farmer who brought in this Suffolk, is very experienced and our phone conversation was brief. We agreed to meet down at the surgery's lambing shed in 15 minutes' time.

Stephen is friendly but quite serious. A man of very few words – unless of course, he's on his specialist subject: his animals. In which case, he could very well talk until the cows, quite literally, come home.

That's what you want, really. As severe as opening up a womb sounds, it really is quite routine for a rural vet, and a bit of chat in the early hours is rarely unwelcome. In all honesty, it can be a little awkward when you're working in the middle of the night and the only other person in the room opts to stay completely silent. The typical shop-talk routines to encourage a bit of conversation over a Caesar might kick off with 'It feels like a big lamb.' This is a vet classic, just to lend the farmer the reassurance that they did the right thing opting to bring the ewe to the practice in the first place. You might then graduate to a 'So, how's lambing going?' Perhaps in this case I'll hazard his response: 'This is one of the first of the year actually.' And then you just hope the chat continues to flow and you don't get the one- or two-word responses that lead you into an awkward conversational cul-de-sac.

Over the years I've got to know a lot of farmers, and farming families, very well. What you generally get is a good conversation between people who are on genuinely quite friendly terms. There's a fair bit of jocular banter too, which could revolve around them bemoaning the price of veterinary treatment, leading me to poke them about the reputation farmers foster in regard to thriftiness.

With many, I'll ask about a former patient or steer to a known favourite topic: 'Dare I ask what happened to the down cow I treated?' or 'Are you getting the results you hoped for with the embryo transfer programme?' Then, as ever, there's always the great Scottish failsafe: the weather. But it is by no means a disaster if someone really is the reticent type, of course; I can go solo on a multitude of topics, a few of which I might even know a little about.

Conversation does more than just pass the time; it helps builds bonds too. You can go out to a farm, complete a job in 20 minutes, and then easily spend another 20 minutes just leaning over your car door, having a chat. We were always taught by the, now retired, senior partners never to short-change any of our customers unless we have an emergency to attend. I'm the kind of person who is happy to chat anyway, but we all see it as very much part of the job. There's the job we actually charge for, and then there's all the free advice that we don't. It's a two-way street: I've learnt plenty from the farmers I've worked with over the years, and they've helped me gain a real insight into their farms, and the farming industry as a whole – which in turn helps me do my job better. All that at the cost of a bit of leaning time, or a cup of tea down in the farmhouse.

The majority of our farms are multi-species, meaning they farm two or more types of animal. Most often it's cattle and sheep, as on Stephen's farm. He and I proceed to chat away about this past autumn. It was a particularly wet one, which saw a bit of a pneumonia problem spread among his calves, so I'm not surprised that the discussion for this Caesar revolves around vaccination options he might want to consider. Thinking about what most other people are doing at three o'clock on a cold morning, perhaps the idea of me engaging in a long chat in a large shed about subjects ranging from agricultural politics to aborted calves – just so I can pass the time while I deliver a lamb – might seem quite bizarre, but it's all very much part of our world.

There is no question that this Suffolk is going to need a Caesar. Not only do I trust Stephen's judgement implicitly, but the ewe has only managed to push the tips of her lamb's sizeable front hooves clear of her vulva and out into open air. The rest of the lamb is trapped firmly inside and nothing they have attempted back at the farm has shifted it a single inch further towards liberation. This lamb is far too big for its mum's pelvis and a Caesar is the best way to save them from each other.

The Suffolk is a large breed, so thankfully we have a hydraulic table to pump the ewe up to a comfortable height for me to work on her. The table and its hydraulics probably get put under greater pressure than almost any other piece of equipment in the surgery, and the classic time to realise that it's not working properly would be right now: in the small hours on the first Caesar of the year. Happily, though, this morning, everything is in fine working order.

Stephen and I lay the ewe on her side. I take up some rope and fasten the back legs in a splayed position, leaving her front end for Stephen to restrain while I work. It is really important that whoever is on the front does a good job of controlling the sheep. You don't want an animal, often in excess of 100kg in weight, throwing itself around during a procedure that involves a sharp blade and an open body cavity.

In the human surgical world, when it comes to a C-section delivery, you'll have a whole team of people working around the mum. Everything in the room is tailored towards that one very important task, and everyone, apart from the mum and the dad or significant other, is a professionally trained and experienced practitioner skilled in facilitating that particular operation. With sheep Caesars, you've just got to assume that a farmer, or shepherd, is naturally up for the task; but that has not always been the case.

Once, I was performing an early-morning Caesar when a farmer suddenly vacated his position by collapsing into the corner of the lambing shed. I was deep into the operation and so I had lost not only the other person in the room but also the sole means of controlling the front end of the sheep, whose womb I was starting to stitch up.

The anaesthesia used is only local, like at the dentist, so the sheep are fully conscious and often kindly offer a substitute for electronic life-sign monitors by moving their legs or trying to sit up. So, the farmer is conked out and slumped against the shed wall, I'm standing with one hand on the sheep and one hand on my stitching needle, and I'm just wondering, *What on earth am I going to do next?*

What if the farmer had just suffered a heart attack? He could have been dead for all I could tell. I definitely needed to give him urgent attention, but on the other hand, this sheep was now only half-restrained and semi-stitched, and my hands were completely covered in its blood and bodily fluid. If it weren't such a serious situation, you could almost be fooled into thinking it was some sort of hidden-camera comedy prank.

I grabbed the front end of the sheep with one hand, lest she leap up, then I spun around the table and managed to nudge him. 'Are you alright?' was the best I could do given the circumstances, but it seemed to do the trick. He was not dead. He was breathing. He stirred a little and then he came around.

'Oh, er,' he groaned, 'I didn't have any breakfast this morning.' He remained seated, propped up by the wall, and I returned to the sheep – which, thankfully, had remained wonderfully well behaved throughout the ordeal.

I resumed my needlework. However, after a lucid couple of minutes the farmer passed out once again. This time I was at least reassured that it was unlikely he was dead. As he slumbered with a concrete wall as his pillow, I quickly wrapped up the stitching. On coming to a second time, I insisted he immediately call his wife; I wasn't going to let him drive home.

As she swept into the shed, the farmer was already back up on his feet and had regained some of his colour. 'Er, didn't have any breakfast …' he began, before being promptly cut off by his wife: 'Don't be giving me that rubbish! You were exactly the same when I gave birth to our son!'

Surgery complete, the ewe, her newborn lamb, the wife and the red-faced farmer were soon all on their way.

Tonight, my chief support is going to do a good job. I know Stephen has seen it all before. This certainly isn't the first occasion we've spent together over a hole in the side of one of his cows or sheep.

With the sheep comfortably on her side, I remove the fleece from her flank with some clippers. It doesn't fall off quite as easily in the midwinter as it will in the later months, heading towards the summer shearing season. When it's warmer, a sheep's fleece is naturally much more ready to shed, but the clippers make light work of it for now. Next, I administer a 'line block' of local anaesthetic with a needle and syringe, effectively numbing the tissue I am about to incise, and I dose her up with penicillin and an anti-inflammatory. Then I scrub up, thoroughly sterilising and scrubbing the freshly shorn flank with disinfectant and water, ensuring there is very little chance of any dirt or bacteria getting into the operating area.

'It's probably the cleanest she's been since she was born!' I quip to Stephen, who is keeping pressure on the ewe's shoulders.

'Probably,' he replies, with a wry smile.

With the ewe now ready to go, I make my final preparations. With sheep Caesars, I usually operate without gloves. With cows, I'll fully cover up, as the blood can dry hard to the skin and be very tough to shift, but with sheep, I much prefer to be able to go in with my bare hands. It's more tactile and I can easily clean myself. The downside, however, is that your hands and arms are left with a persistent aroma afterwards, even once you've washed them thoroughly. They basically smell of mutton, and in the heart of lambing time that smell becomes pretty much my permanent eau de parfum. My wife eats lots of goat's cheese at home, and honestly, I can't go near the stuff. Goats and sheep may be different species, but the 'sheepy' smell of that cheese is all too familiar to my nose, and one whiff triggers a singularly unpalatable thought: *Sheep Caesars.*

I make what I hope will be a lamb-sized horizontal incision along the lower edge of the Suffolk's side, through the skin, muscle and peritoneum (the thin tissue lining the sheep's abdominal cavity). Once I penetrate this, a little fluid immediately spills out alongside a portion of her intestine. Gently, I replace the intestinal loop within the cavity, and, with my fingers functioning as eyes, I feel for the womb, or uterus, and manipulate it out of the abdominal incision. Unsurprisingly, given the size of the lamb inside it, the womb is unmissable, and currently vying with the sheep's capacious forestomach as the largest abdominal organ.

The uterus is Y-shaped, not too dissimilar to a ram's horns in appearance, and one of those horns is fit to burst. Now in position, I use a pair of scissors to make an incision through the wall of the uterus. I prefer scissors over the scalpel for this cut as, simply, I don't want to risk damaging the unborn lamb in any way. The incision reveals a pair of back legs covered in shiny placental membranes. I break through these and a rush of slimy fluid vents onto the table, my waterproofs and the floor. I'm now able to grip the legs and ease them through the gap I've created, before the rest of what is a real lump of a lamb follows with one final firm but gentle pull.

In the shelter of our lambing shed, in the smallest hours of the morning, I suspend Stephen's newest flock member by its back legs with one hand, and wipe the amniotic goo covering its mouth with the other. It has been a very swift and fruitful job, and with a couple of brisk rubs to the chest, the lamb soon splutters, forcing the first breaths of fresh air down into its tiny lungs.

Half an hour later, I am completely alone. The stitching was routine and the ewe, the farmer and their larger-than-average lamb have all made their way safely back to the farm. The gory stuff – the blood and all the bodily fluids from the operation – had pooled up over the metal table and flowed down onto the floor. I slooshed down the area and then cleaned myself before ensuring everything was ready to go again for when the next animal graces the shed.

It doesn't matter how many times you do it. That feeling of delivering a new life into the world never gets old; and the first of a new year is always special.

Chapter Four

A Prolapse in Deep Snow

January rolled forward with routine operations on the pet side of the practice. The vets in the field were out doing a bit of large-animal testing, mostly cattle for tuberculosis, and tending to numerous lame cows with foot conditions, before Burns Night came around at the month's end.

Burns Night celebrates Scotland's own national bard, the great poet Robert Burns, who lived, worked and died in the eighteenth century. His works are famous worldwide for making cultural and political comment, often quite bluntly, and his New Year's ode 'Auld Lang Syne' is among the most widely sung folk songs in the Scots language. Each year on January 25th, Scots mark the anniversary of his birth by gathering with friends to enjoy a hearty dinner of haggis, neeps (swede) and tatties. Dramatic speeches are delivered in tribute to the great bard, along with multiple toasts and enthusiastic recitals of some of his most treasured poems and songs.

It might become a little riotous or crude at times, but along with the haggis, the tongue is also often firmly in the cheek, and it is a great way of closing the opening month of the year. My fellow director, Ken, has a reputation for a belting Burns speech, and is often booked up for community Burns Nights well in advance of the twenty-fifth.

This January was one to endure, rather than enjoy. The stunning winter days were very few and far between. It was mostly wet, windy and (you guessed it) dreich, with only a few scattered snowfalls. It was a far cry from the snow-filled Januarys that used to consistently come to Caithness a few decades ago. Our elderly inhabitants can even recall a handful of the infamously severe winters. Cars were left stranded and there was a regrettable loss of life on the 'braes', the slopes, at Berriedale. An old farmer told me that conditions were once so severe that food parcels were dropped from aircraft, and I even remember being told the story of a women's hosiery salesman who, trapped by deep snow in his potential tomb of a vehicle, fought off the fatal cold by layering himself up with all the tights and stockings he had intended for sale.

As a child – albeit one much further south in Lancashire – I, too, can remember having quite a few big snow days. Back then, the snowdrifts were often so deep we could actually build caves in them. My brothers and I would stay out sledging until we couldn't feel our feet, and our springer spaniel would leap around with huge dangly balls of snow that had developed in place of her great floppy ears.

Winters are not what they used to be. Increasingly, they seem to be becoming warmer and wetter. While climate change may be an issue we all need to face, the changing prevalence of some diseases can bring particular challenges to vets and animal owners.

Another twist to add spice to winter scenarios is our coastal location. With modern cars displaying the external air temperature,

I have noticed on many calls that a tropical 0 degrees in Thurso can drop to minus 3 or 4 by the time I approach a farm less than ten miles inland. You must be wary of a false sense of security on such occasions. What may be a light sprinkling of snow in the town can easily become significantly deeper layers of ice or snow in the countryside, where the roads are often much more treacherous.

During my time in Caithness we have had only a few notable years where a deep and heavy snowfall managed to cover both town and country. An incident while on call has fixed such a night in my mind indelibly. I can't remember there being a worse night of snow in all of my time up here.

One February day during my early years at the practice, the snow fell ceaselessly and the conditions were just right to make it really stick. We knew from weather warnings that we were in for a bad spell, but, in the comfort of the surgery and with a home in town, I don't remember being too worried.

Here in Thurso the vets operate on a first and second on-call system. This is essential to cope with the workload, particularly at busy times of year. The first on-call vet attends to the calls as they arise and the second is only needed when consecutive emergencies occur, or if help is required for a more complex job. Bridget, a senior colleague, was first on call that night, and as her second, I was hoping for a cosy night in.

Soon after midnight our home phone rang. The practice phone line is diverted to our house out of hours, so that wasn't a huge surprise, but as I answered it, the farmer on the line explained that one of his cows was suffering from a 'bed-out'. This was not, I'm afraid to say, an incident involving a large animal merely refusing to remain in its sleeping quarters. To vets, a bed-out is a uterine prolapse, meaning, after this cow had successfully birthed her calf, her womb had followed it out and was now dangling from her back end.

It was a genuine emergency. Without prompt attention, the cow would die.

Getting woken up by the phone is never pleasant, but it's a lot easier when I know I can send another vet out into the cold before returning my head to my pillow. I called Bridget with the news of the prolapse, but her response was not what I wanted to hear. She had recently moved out of town and bought a farm on which to keep her horses. The snow there, she explained, was now so deep that she wouldn't even make it down her farm track, let alone negotiate the treacherous main roads to reach the farm in question.

In town, where the sea air and moving traffic had kept the snow level at bay, it appeared I was in a much better location to respond to the call. I peeled myself from my bed, got dressed and cleared the snow from the car. Any foot-dragging soon disappeared into the freezing midnight sky. This was a critical situation for the farmer and his cow, and I felt a little buzz of excitement as I realised that I was the only one in a position to resolve it.

My car made it to the edge of town with relative ease considering the severity of the conditions, but then, as I approached the point where the road headed to open country, I came across something I had never seen before and have not stumbled across since: a large signpost cut across my half of the road. It was a police roadblock.

Use of the road out of town was prohibited due to the snowfall. I hovered in my car, staring at the sign. What would I do? I had a cow that needed immediate veterinary attention but a roadblock in front of me telling me to go absolutely no further. There were no police officers around to ask for advice; they probably had more sense than to stay out in the cold.

Could I really fly in the face of a clear police notice? I might save a cow, but would I then be arrested? I could see that the two-laned road ahead had one lane reasonably clear as it led away, but would it remain clear as I progressed further inland? The farm was halfway down the bleak and windswept Causeway Mire. Was the sign indicating that the road was totally impassable? What if I slid off into a ditch and got stuck for hours, or even days, without the traditional supply of stockings or tights to clothe myself?

I thought of the reason for the call. It wasn't some routine visit that could be put off; it was life or death. I had no option but to attempt to get there. I persuaded myself that the roadblock was advisory, or that at least I would be forgiven for bypassing it under the circumstances.

As I cautiously pulled out of Thurso, the normally two-laned road continued as a one-laned trench. Walls of snow, pushed up by the last pass of the snowplough, towered on each side of the car, and regular small drifts, flurries and patches of snow fell right across my path. I kept what I hoped was a safe but steady speed, reasoning that the sensible thing would be to push on and keep the wheels straight. Breaking or turning felt like a very good way to skid off the road completely. I was tense and on edge as I drove, yet I'll admit to a sense of invigoration: *I'm making progress, I'm actually getting there!*

I managed the turn-off onto the great Causeway Mire with no loss of traction, but I anticipated the conditions might very well be set to worsen the deeper inland I travelled. By this point,

I was pretty much fully committed. There was no way I could have turned the car around there, even if I had wanted to.

Suddenly, there were flashing lights ahead. It had crossed my mind that if I met anything coming from the opposite direction then we would both be snookered, trapped in our one-laned trench, but it turned out that this was a real beacon of hope: the orange flashing light of the snowplough, working out here through the night, and clearing the road once more.

As the only vehicle fully capable of comfortably penetrating these conditions, it quickly ploughed through beside me and came to a halt. The window of the cab wound down and I met a face clearly poised to give me both barrels. Before I could get any words out, the stern-faced driver unleashed, 'What on earth are you doing out here, you idiot?!' I quickly explained I was a vet on an emergency call, and his countenance changed immediately. He motioned that the road was now fully clear behind him and sent me on my way.

As promised by the plough driver, the remainder of the trip was much easier and I arrived at the farm to find, thankfully, a straightforward bed-out; believe me, they aren't always. The cow was still standing, which is always a good sign. I gave a caudal epidural – an injection of local anaesthetic into the spine where the tail joins the body – to numb the rear end of the cow. The epidural is more than just a painkiller. Any mother will tell you that the instinctive desire to push when in labour is very hard to consciously override. It had caused the cow to thrust out both her calf and then her womb, but this urge would be effectively turned off by the epidural. Without this precision-placed injection, any attempt by me to push her inverted womb back through her birth canal would have immediately stimulated the same reflex. Inevitably, a cow can push harder than a vet, and so there is a real danger of fingers or a fist shooting through the tissue of the womb and creating a tear. The epidural is a wondrous blessing, abolishing the irresistible urge to push and allowing a vet to crack on with their work unimpeded.

I successfully replaced the womb into the belly of the cow and stitched the vulva as a security measure to dissuade her from repeat-offending while her body settled down to its normal rhythm over the following few days.

In the small hours of the morning, I rolled back down the hill towards my town. The snowplough had done its job and the journey home wasn't anything like as dramatic as the outbound adventure. This time there was a policeman stationed at the road-block, which I was now, very obviously, on the wrong side of.

I slowed and nervously lowered my window. 'The road's now clear behind me and along the Cazziemire,' is all I said. He didn't make a grab for his handcuffs; I was safe! I added no further backstory, but drove on quickly, taking pleasure in the bemused expression etched across his face, which was clearly displaying the question 'Where did *he* come from?'

In reality, no vehicle other than a snowplough had the right to make it out and back again in such deep snow, but these are the decisions we sometimes have to take as Highland vets.

I made it home for a few hours of rest and warmth before the day's work started once again.

Chapter Five

Valentine's at the Vets

February 14th. Valentine's Day at the practice.

I can't say I'm hugely sold on the idea of the day itself. Fun at school, perhaps, but if I needed a special prescribed day to tell my wife I loved her it would be fair to wonder whether our marriage was in trouble! How much better to offer a romantic gesture when she's not expecting it and away from the commercialism of the global event. Okay, I admit to buying a rose for our first Valentine's Day, when our relationship was embryonic, but my withering excuse for a flower was outdone by another admirer, who left Jennifer a specimen worthy to win at the Chelsea Flower Show. Scoundrel!

I suppose I'd better also own up to entering into the cheesiness of the day in more recent years. I orchestrated a romantic photo of Milis, our cute Labrador puppy, offering a big Valentine's heart to Shadow, the young Lab of our niece, whom she had met fleetingly a few weeks earlier at Christmas. Of course, we kept them from the mistletoe, we couldn't risk them chewing on it. It appeared to be a case of love at first sniff. However, as you might expect, it turned out it was only puppy love.

The sentiment, though, of expressing affection and gratitude to our loved ones, certainly isn't lost on me. I've been very happily married to Jennifer for almost 30 years and, although it may be a bit of a cliché, she's always been a pillar of strength in my life.

We first met at Pollock Halls, one of the main University of Edinburgh halls of residence. It was 1988 and Jennifer and I were both first years – freshers. Vet students are renowned for being cliquey; we tend to stick together and socialise within the faculty. Many vet–vet romances sprang up in my cohort, but Jennifer was on a different course, so it was a stroke of providence that we met at all.

During the first day of our first year, one of my soon-to-be friends, Alison, had wandered around Pollock Halls looking for other fresher vet students to talk to. Pretty soon she'd gathered a small group of us, but she'd also bumped into Jennifer on her travels and they'd hit it off immediately.

What can I say really? I fancied Jennifer from the very first time we met, but we didn't start going out until the second term. She was undeniably pretty, with a warm smile and friendly blue eyes. She also possessed a head of light brown hair with a distinctive wave in it. I think it was a hangover from a proper eighties perm that she'd sported the previous year – and which triggered a family member to comment, 'You look like you've been dragged through a hedge backwards!' – but for some reason it all added to the attraction for me.

Jennifer recalls her first impression of me. I was tanned, with sun-bleached hair, and was attired in vivid clothing, displaying what she describes as an 'interesting' sense of colour coordination. She presumed, excitedly, that I must have been some kind of exotic continental smoothie, but was disappointed when my accent gave me away and she discovered I'd been bronzed on my gap year in Africa, and that I'd inherited colour blindness from my grandfather.

Jennifer remained in our little group of vets and we all social-ised a lot together, but pretty soon she and I were finding ourselves engineering excuses to be alone. The most obvious example was how Jennifer would ask me to help with her physics homework. Once I knew her better, it was apparent that this had all been a ruse. She had needed no help, at least not from me. Jennifer is exceptionally bright; if we'd been at school together, she would no doubt have annoyed me by always getting better marks. She graduated with a first-class honours degree in chemistry and was among the top students in her year, but her feigned struggles did give us an excuse to spend time together until it became so appar-ent to everyone that excuses were no longer needed.

University days ticked on and our relationship grew ever stronger; soon we knew we wanted to be together for good. One blustery, grey spring day during our third year at university, with the promise of a Mars bar on reaching the top, I persuaded Jennifer to climb Arthur's Seat – the big volcanic rock overlook-ing Edinburgh and, more immediately, Pollock Halls. I dropped to one knee and Jennifer presumed I was finding the Mars bar in my rucksack. But instead, with a ring I'd been hiding in my sock drawer, I proposed and received a very surprised and enthusiastic yes as the clouds parted and rays of sunshine cast down upon us (as my best man so poetically described the events in his wedding speech). We thought at that point we would wed after my gradu-ation. Jennifer was to graduate after her four-year course, but my veterinary degree was always scheduled to run for another year.

Then we thought, *Why wait?* and so we arranged it all for a year earlier than we'd planned.

Even back in the nineties, that might have seemed a little rushed or old-fashioned, but for us, the most important thing was that we were together; everything else could just work around that. I do remember feeling the vibes that others thought I should graduate before wedlock. 'Getting married now is ridiculous! You're far too young!' insisted a medical school friend. Like so many other peers, he went on to fall in love and marry only a few years later; it just all happened a bit sooner for Jennifer and me. Of course, the benefit of having a wife to look after me during my finals hadn't crossed my mind, though I'll admit it was a pleasant bonus.

I feel so blessed to have married Jennifer. She has been wonderfully supportive throughout my life and career. She was a full-time mum when our children were really young but, once they were both in school, she retrained and gained a post-graduate teaching qualification. Now she has been a primary school teacher for over 15 years, but in those early years she effectively juggled all the challenges of her work, her training and the needs of our children against the demands of my job, with all its anti-social hours and unscheduled emergency call-outs. She has put up with so much on account of my chosen career.

Jennifer has actually been employed by the practice as an out-of-hours telephonist since before she became a teacher. Whenever I'm either first or second on-call, the practice phone line is diverted to our house. For many years she has been responsible for waking up vets in the middle of the night, or ruining their social functions, or disturbing them at a critical point in the film they were watching. Fielding the calls is a stressful job when they are flooding in at peak season in spring, and her long suffering in the face of numerous shooting-the-messenger comments from grumpy vets (often me) is a real testament to her strength of character. Even today, she is still the point of contact whenever I'm on duty out of hours. It's a habit that has never died; it's become a way of life.

No matter what, I can look back on everything we've achieved together through three decades of happy marriage and confidently say that pair of apparently naive twenty-somethings was right all along.

Veterinary medicine has a way of drawing lovers together. For example, Scye and Mey are two sisters from our locality. During my time up here, they went off in turn to the vet school at the University of Edinburgh and did much of their required practical placement with us. At university they met a couple of eligible young men: Tom, now a Thurso vet, and Pete, who became one of our directors at the Wick surgery. Tom and Pete are now married to Scye and Mey respectively. As I said, vets can be cliquey!

We have also, naturally, seen romances bloom within the surgery itself. The most obvious of which involved Ken, one of our vets, and Catherine, who was our head nurse.

I remember once needing to catch an urgent word with Ken but for some reason I couldn't raise him on the phone. I was fairly sure he was at home so I decided to call past his house. I tried to act unsurprised to find that Catherine was there too. Nothing had ever been mentioned about them being together, at least not to me.

I didn't say anything, of course. I just sat and chatted about the topic in hand, and then didn't mention anything to others about what was quite rightly their private life. I could understand why they might want to maintain discretion, especially in the early days of their relationship.

However, not too long after that, Ken was kicked in the head by a horse and rushed to hospital. Getting kicked by animals is something he has since turned into a new sport; his most recent trip to A&E was at the hands (or rather hooves) of a young bullock. However, on that first occasion, I was in the operating room with Catherine when we got the news, and others were working within earshot. Not wanting to blow their privacy and make it blindingly obvious to the rest of the staff that I knew they were an item, I resorted to exaggerated facial expressions and flicks of my head to try to persuade her that she should get herself over to the hospital.

It's quite funny looking back at it all now. I have since come to realise that I am often the last to learn of the twists and turns of the private affairs of our staff and clients, and so perhaps, with hindsight, my discretion may have been unnecessary. I'm very happy to report that Ken's head still functions well despite his trauma and that he and Catherine are still very much together and now have a couple of young children.

The other obvious romance was between vet Fiona and one of our local farmers. Kenneth was a client whose family farm I had been visiting since he was a teenager. Years later when Fiona arrived in Caithness as a newly qualified vet, she set out to impress our farmers with her veterinary skills, but without trying, managed to make an impression on Kenneth in a totally different way. After a period of wooing, he won her over. Their wedding, at Fiona's hometown further south, felt like a *Highland Vet* weekend break.

They must have been married for about 10 years now, also with young kids.

It's not really that surprising that strong relationships have formed through working alongside each other. We work closely with people, often in highly pressurised situations, and it is through sharing the ups and downs of a job like ours that, when tensions subside, lasting friendships are forged and even true love can be kindled.

Striking the balance between work and family life is not easy. Jennifer, I'm sure, would say that most of the time the balance has definitely been tipped too far in favour of my work. The one saving grace is that I do live near the surgery, so when on call I have at least been able to go in, do the work, and get home for a meal or a break before the phone rings again. But there are other times when a call-out takes me away from Thurso, or its nature is just a lot more serious and committing. Those are the times when social engagements, birthdays, school plays, sports days, nights out and plans with friends can be missed. It was a fact that the producers of *The Highland Vet* picked up on in the very first episode they shot with me.

In my maiden sequence for the series, I'm found on a farm, engaged in an absolute classic vet story. 'I don't think there is anything finer than being out in the middle of the Highlands lathering yourself up for a surgical procedure on a cow,' I comment to camera, as I prepare to conduct a Caesar on a hefty Limousin-cross heifer. It was actually mid-December, so not the traditional spring calving season by any stretch. This young cow had fallen pregnant after jumping a wall and meeting up with a bull at a time far earlier than the farmer had planned.

The producers had identified a quirky side story whereby I had needed to get the surgery wrapped up so I could get home and keep a date with my wife. Funnily enough, they also featured a shot of an old tea tray that was holding all my surgical instruments at the time. Why use such a battered and faded item? Well, it still does the job perfectly, but more than that, it has sentimental value. Jennifer had in fact used it to bring me tea back in our university days.

The segment finishes with the successful caesarean birth of the cow's healthy, but quite large, calf, and then it picks up again with me at my 'date', which happened to be our regular ballroom dancing class. I didn't think a huge amount of it at the time, but since the programme aired, more than one farmer has quipped, 'So, Guy, are you in a rush to get back for your dancing?'

Sometimes, though, events conspire to make sure you definitely don't make the date. Quite a few years ago, one of our nursing assistants was getting married. I was on call that weekend, so it was always going to be a bit touch-and-go as to whether I would make it to the ceremony or the reception, or both, or neither. Jennifer and I had managed to make it together to the church ceremony as planned, but, as it so often goes, that evening I was indeed called away on an emergency. Quite extraordinarily, though, it was actually the dog of an important guest at the wedding. Ann, the bride's auntie, had a springer spaniel which had suddenly started fitting dangerously. Fits in dogs are, unfortunately, not uncommon, and most are caused by what we vets would categorise as 'idiopathic epilepsy': an inherited disorder which we don't really know the root cause of.

We use the word 'fit' interchangeably with the more medical term 'seizure'. Other possible causes of fits in dogs include head trauma, brain tumours, certain infections, toxins, even liver disease or other outside-of-the-brain disorders, but the unifying factor in all seizures is that they cause a considerable disturbance to normal brain function. A seizure is an unpredictable and abnormal firing of a small portion of nerve tissue within the brain that causes an overwhelming cascade of electrical activity and release of brain signalling chemicals known as neurotransmitters. Overactivity in parts of the brain engulfed by this avalanche can present outwardly in many ways, often including quite violent involuntary movements and muscle spasms.

Fits can affect dogs young and old, and certain breeds, such as Border collies and beagles, are more vulnerable than others to the idiopathic form, which usually presents itself at a young age. One or two very occasional fits may not be a huge concern. If they do become more frequent, though, they can usually be controlled well with regular medication that the owners can easily give their animal at home. It's stressful to watch a dog fitting, and owners will commonly phone in a real panic. Thankfully most seizures are short-lived, and normality soon resumes. The aim of treatment is to reduce the frequency and severity of the fits or, if you're lucky, to eliminate them.

A very worrying problem arrives when a dog has either a prolonged fit, lasting five minutes or more with no sign of it abating, or if several fits occur in a row. For us as vets these cases can be quite challenging. It's not just the fits themselves – the tremors in the muscles, the uncontrollable jerking of the body and paddling of the legs, sometimes the foaming at the mouth, eye-rolling, or even the passing of urine and faeces – it's the injury that all that excessive electrical activity is doing to their brain. Ultimately, long-term, frequent fitting could start to cause an animal irreparable brain damage.

When a badly fitting dog is hospitalised, we place an intra-venous (IV) line, which can then be used to inject appropriate anti-fitting medication straight into the dog's bloodstream. Then, as the medication wears off, we need to monitor very closely in case the dog lapses into fitting again. With Auntie Ann's springer, it was very quickly apparent that I was going to have to monitor her exceptionally closely at the surgery. When she was brought in, she seemed to be either fitting or about to fit, and even after I'd dosed her with medication, she was quite quickly dropping back into a seizure state again.

Jennifer, who was now an unattached plus-one at the wedding reception, was texting me to ask if I was likely to make it back to the party with the rest of the veterinary staff. I explained that I would not only miss the party but would likely have to remain with the dog throughout the night. On hearing this, Ann herself declared, 'Well, if he's not making the party because he's looking after my dog, I'm not having him miss out on the meal.' She marched into the hotel's kitchen and insisted that a takeaway meal be plated up. After Jennifer delivered it to me at the surgery, I sent her back to the fun; I was somewhat preoccupied and there was no point both of us missing out on the celebration.

The spaniel exhausted me with a night of intensive monitoring and treatment. Thankfully, she eventually recovered, but it had taken a lot out of both me and her. A couple of years ago, the same thing actually happened to me all over again, although with no wedding to get to on this occasion. I recalled just how uncomfortable the night had been for me the last time around, and made the discovery that if you take our veterinary bedding – the thick, fluffy fabric mats we have to keep our animals comfortable – and then pile them three or four beds thick on the kennel room floor, you can actually catch a short period of sleep before the patient wakes you up with another seizure.

These days we have a noise-sensitive camera that connects to the Wi-Fi, not dissimilar to the baby monitors many new parents have in their homes. The camera allows us to see and hear the patients in the kennel area without having to actually sleep on the floor next to them. Nonetheless, the imperative to be on hand as quickly as possible is still the same, and there is no substitute for physically attending an animal, no matter the time of day or night and regardless of the plans you might have had elsewhere.

One thing is for sure: when my wife wakes up and I'm not there in the night, I'm pretty certain to be found either down at the practice or out on a farm, working on an emergency call-out. Sometimes I'll even lie awake at night when I'm not on call, reflecting obsessively on a difficult case I dealt with that day. If the animal was admitted for overnight care, rather than wake up the on-call vet with my concerns, I've occasionally made the decision to go down to the practice to check how it's doing. Poor Jennifer. She used to tell me off about it, reminding me that when I'm *not* on call, it's really *not* my job, but she's since learnt to just accept that part of my character. Besides, I'm more likely to nod off again if I've checked and know that all is well.

Chapter Six

All Creatures Small and Smaller

Winter has really had us firmly in its talons this year. Usually, as we break the back of February, we'll get small signs that spring might just be waiting around the corner: a gentle easing of the cold, perhaps a few days with double-digit temperatures, and then the very earliest of the springtime flowers puncturing the topsoil with their green shoots.

Not this winter, though.

January blended indistinguishably into February, and it remained steadfastly damp and miserable outside. The winter coats stayed firmly on our backs, and the all-weather tyres were a must to keep us vets safe when out on our calls.

No matter what the weather or season, our run of jobs in the small-animal wing of the practice trundles forward without let-up. Covid-19 restrictions reduced routine work in the early part of the year, such as vaccinations and neutering, but animals still fell ill or injured themselves and couldn't be left to suffer. Some surgery was necessary; for example, I dealt with a few cruciate ligament injuries, which are a frequent cause of lameness in dogs. Veterinary staples continued in the form of nasty cat bite abscesses. (Cats effectively inoculate their adversary with a bacterial cocktail residing on their fangs; it's a gruesome but strangely satisfying task to empty out the pus.) Medical disorders continued to require investigation, the classic example being 'I've got a temperature but I'm going to let you work out why the hard way.' Weight loss or excessive thirst are other presenting signs that are always best followed through to unearth the root cause. Then, of course, there were dogs causing havoc in their intestines by eating things they shouldn't have.

Cats are usually much more discerning about what they put in their mouths, but as winter made its earliest attempt to progress into spring, I dealt with the more unusual case of a cat eating a substance which was certainly not recommended as part of its ordinary diet. To be fair, it wasn't as if this cat, a six-year-old called Jess, had done it deliberately. Perhaps while investigating innocently, she brushed up against a vase filled with lilies, which then deposited their pollen all over her fur. Cats are naturally fastidious when it comes to the state of their coats, so Jess proceeded to lick herself clean and, in doing so, swallowed the dusty orange lily pollen.

It all sounds fairly innocuous, until you realise that some lilies are extremely toxic if ingested by animals, including humans. The level of toxicity varies depending on the lily species and the animal species eating it. For cats, though, any lily in the true lily or daylily families can be potentially fatal. It's not just the pollen; the entire lily plant is toxic from the stem to the leaves, from the petals to even the water in the vase. If just a small amount of a toxic lily enters a cat's system and is left untreated, it could actually cause total kidney failure and thus prove fatal within days.

The extreme reaction cats have is not simply explained by the fact that they are so much smaller than dogs or people. Cats can be quirky. It seems they are particularly sensitive to lily poison. Another quirk is that the emetic drug we use to make a dog sick is not really recommended nor all that effective in cats.

So, what we use as the first port of call for inducing vomiting in cats is a sedative drug called xylazine, which is well known for its side effect of making them queasy. The hope was that after I injected Jess with xylazine, she would throw up and thus effectively clear her stomach of the toxic pollen. Of course, when it came to Jess that day, Murphy's Law kicked in, whereby I guarantee you now, had I wanted to simply sedate her, she would have been sick, but when I wanted her to be sick, she became sedated without vomiting!

It took a good half hour for Jess to come around from her, essentially pointless, sleep, before I could then attempt plan B. This came in the form of good old-fashioned soda crystals. Now, this is not something you want to ever attempt with your pets at home as you need to be sure you use the right type, but soda crystals can be used as an effective emetic for both dogs and cats. I placed a couple of crystals on the back of Jess's tongue. We waited. Nothing, just drooling. I administered another dose of crystals and waited once more: again, nothing but sticky saliva.

By this point I was starting to get more than just a little concerned. There are only so many soda crystals you can give a cat before you really have to consider the possibility that you're now just risking poisoning it with something else. So here was Jess, still seemingly untroubled by the crystals, the xylazine, or, apparently, the lily pollen.

The real problem was that, for as long as I failed to make Jess vomit, the deeper the toxins from the lily pollen would work their way into her system, before ultimately they began attacking her kidneys. Thankfully, her owner had brought Jess into us the moment he'd realised she'd consumed the pollen, so we knew we had a small buffer zone with respect to timing.

If only she would vomit! I thought, then I could have possibly sent her home straight away. But Jess was being frustratingly non-compliant, and time was ticking on.

You might think the next obvious move would be a stomach pump, but that's far from straightforward. Cats tend to swallow their food in chunks after little, if any, chewing. The stomach slowly mushes up these chunks and moves the resulting soup into the intestines. Before this happens, these pieces – up to a centimetre across – remain in the stomach. The size of the tube you can pass into a cat's stomach has a bore nowhere near big enough to suck out such large chunks, so it was useful to know whether her stomach was full of food before proceeding.

I X-rayed Jess and, sure enough, discovered a belly full of breakfast. Given what was at stake, I decided a stomach wash-out was still worth a go. With her under anaesthetic, I flushed a little fluid into her stomach and then tried sucking the contents back up the tube.

That was pretty unrewarding too. A hat-trick! Two attempts to make her vomit and one effort at siphoning out the poison; all had failed. I was finding it hard to hide my frustration from the TV camera following the case. The only option left to me, if I was intent on physically removing the pollen, was to open the stomach surgically and empty it myself. I think most vets would agree this would have been an excessive step and so I dismissed it. I opted instead for aggressive intravenous fluid therapy. We placed a drip line into Jess's vein and kept it flowing at a high rate. In very simple terms we were diluting the toxin as it entered her bloodstream and flushing it out through the kidneys, thus hoping it wouldn't linger at a level that might cause organ failure.

We kept Jess in for 48 hours and rechecked her kidney function tests. What a relief! Despite all the setbacks, we found them to be healthy and fully functional, and so finally, we sent her home. She'd probably been wondering what all the fuss was about. Hours of hassle, days of worry, all because this cat simply refused to throw up.

Pretty as lilies may be, I'd advise cat owners to be cautious about ornamenting their houses with them, especially until the veterinary pharmaceutical industry comes up with a gold-standard drug that's certain to make a poisoned cat vomit without undue side effects.

The Highland Vet series has featured all kinds of small-pet stories from across the spectrum of wee species that we see. Some of the more memorable ones for our audience included a guinea pig with a giant cyst, the contents of which were splendidly described by the owner as looking like 'cottage cheese mixed with haggis'; the castration of a whole family of ferrets, calmed before the procedure by an irresistible concoction of fish oils coated on their cage bars for them to lick off; and an unusual pet in an Indian Runner duck that had ended up on the losing side of a fight with his friends. Vets often put such animals under the bracket 'exotics', although it's true a gecko seems to fit that description far better than a rabbit.

Our dogs and cats are so frequent as customers to the small-animal wing, and so popular as pets, that they provide us with many fantastic stories. But there are also many more little creatures gracing our door: everything from hamsters to mice, rats and gerbils; and from small birds such as budgies to cockatiels, pigeons and parrots.

Speaking generally about pets of any kind, there really are more coming to us now than in years gone by. Certainly, during my time in Thurso, I've seen a very definite upward trend in our companion animal workload, which is vying for our attention with farm animal work more than ever before. There are even some serious plans this year to extend the practice building just to accommodate the sheer volume of smaller animals we are now treating throughout the year.

In terms of working on the very smallest of pets, we're probably thinking along the lines of removing tumours from Siberian hamsters, which weigh little more than a few pound coins. A real challenge with mice or hamsters is the handling of them. I've been left with a bleeding finger on more than one occasion. Of course, you learn the tricks of the trade to minimise such risks, but caution, it can be tempting to 'scruff' them by pinching the skin of the neck so you don't get bitten; yet pinch too hard and you actually risk popping their eyes clean out.

Small exotics can be anaesthetised with gas alone, but therein probably lies one of our big stresses in the small-animal wing: the risk of an anaesthetic-related death increases substantially among these smallest of creatures, especially if they are older or particularly unwell. It's a real catch-22 situation. If an animal requires an operation, then it is likely to require an anaesthetic; opting out of that means opting out of the operation as well. It is always a case of weighing the risk of death from the procedure against the benefit attained if all goes well. This is a judgement call and will depend on how serious the condition is: a no-brainer if the animal is suffering, but in some cases it may be best to leave well alone.

A case in point came along this season with Button the budgie. He arrived with a very nasty growth on the underside of his wing. It may have been tumorous, though perhaps was more likely to be a feather cyst – a messy swelling in a feather follicle. He was in his early teens, which, given pet budgies usually only live between five and eight years, made him positively ancient. On examination, it was clear that the cyst was becoming problematic; there was also evidence of self-trauma. Birds can take a notion to peck at abnormal or irritated areas and make them much worse, causing infection or bleeding.

The risk of leaving it was weighed against the risk of surgery. With the owner in the loop, we decided to put Button under anaesthetic. I removed the cyst as quickly as I possibly could, but very sadly, he didn't come round. We had believed that circumstances were driving us to step onto the tightrope of avian anaesthesia, because Button's quality of life could have improved significantly had he pulled through.

There is no getting away from the fact that, in relation to other species we deal with, birds are particularly at risk from anaesthetic-related deaths. But I don't want readers to think the risk of a poor outcome is always high and refuse a required procedure on their bird without discussing all the pros and cons. Like Button, if something needs surgery, discuss it with your vet.

A big part of the problem with birds is that their systems are susceptible to stress. Even without anaesthesia, something as routine as trimming a budgie's nails has been known to stress the delicate creature to the point of a heart attack. However, later on this same season, the cameras captured that hoped-for outcome with another truly dire case. A lady who dedicates her life to caring for abandoned and mistreated animals arrived with her pet chicken, Dixie, which had one of the most severe cases of 'bumblefoot' I have ever seen.

Bumblefoot – or ulcerative pododermatitis, to give its medical name – is a fairly common bacterial infection and inflammatory reaction that can occur on the feet of rodents, rabbits and, as in Dixie's case, birds. The British Hen Welfare Trust describes it as creating the appearance of a chicken wearing 'overlarge carpet slippers', such is the lumpen and swollen presentation of the feet. It is caused by the infection of a wound or small abrasion on the sole of the foot. The foot becomes swollen and inflamed and, all too soon, the infection can progress to the deeper tissues, leading to pus formation and death of the tissue in that region, known as necrosis.

What had happened with Dixie, though, was that the disease had advanced still further. Necrosis had indeed set in, evidenced by the horrid black-brown area on the sole of her foot, but the infection had moved on even beyond that. X-ray showed she now had osteomyelitis – infection in the bone – a dreaded condition because, whatever the species, antibiotics seldom work on it. Frequently the only option is to surgically remove the infected bone.

We were forced into another dance with the anaesthetic dilemma, but the condition was sore to the extent that we had to choose either euthanasia or surgery. Oddly, up against the wall like this, the decision was so much easier. As ever, all the risks and potential outcomes were presented to Dixie's owner, as part of the informed consent process we go through with everyone, and then we proceeded to surgery.

I ended up amputating a toe and removing large chunks of infected bone, and on that occasion, I was relieved to return the bird to the follow-up care of her owner after a smooth and uneventful anaesthetic.

To anesthetise something like a mouse, we will place it in a specialised small-animal anaesthetic chamber. Such containers used to be improvised from sandwich boxes, but nowadays specially designed chambers are available (though they still often look like glorified sandwich boxes). We introduce a mix of oxygen and anaesthetic gas and then, once the mini pet is unconscious, we remove it from the chamber and use a tiny gas mask adapted for petite faces in order to maintain the delivery of the anaesthetic throughout the procedure.

For operating, we have a set of minuscule tools called an eye kit, which is ostensibly for delicate operations on eyes but is equally useful on our more diminutive customers because all the instruments look like baby versions of their normal counterparts: a little pair of scissors, plus finer tweezers, forceps, and needle holders. Additionally, we even have a specialist rodent gag for examining the oral cavity of (oddly enough) rodents and rabbits. The rodent gag was first seen in *The Highland Vet* series when vet Bridget lanced and drained a large abscess on the nose of a rabbit called Buddy, commenting, as she squeezed, 'The trouble with rabbits is they tend to have very thick pus.' The viscosity of its pus, though, is by no means the most peculiar curiosity a rabbit's body throws up.

Rabbits, particularly in the wild, have a diet predominantly made up of grass. We humans would be unable to live exclusively on grass as our gut is unable to digest the cellulose contained within it. Cellulose helps give plants rigidity and structure, but to us it's just undigestible fibre. Indeed, all plant species we eat contain cellulose, but it comes alongside many other nutrients that are beneficial to us; the stuff we can't digest goes through as the all-important roughage. So, for animals that can survive on grass, it is logical to reason that they must have a different gut system to us, one which can derive nutritional value from cellulose.

Take a cow for example. The grass it eats goes into a stomach made up of four distinct compartments. It is convenient to consider the first two of these together as one enormous fermentation vat where the grass arrives after being chewed and swallowed. In this vat reside millions of microscopic organisms such as bacteria, which produce enzymes that can digest cellulose – in other words, break it down so that the products can then be used by the host: the cow.

Portions of the more solid contents of the first compartment are frequently regurgitated back up into the mouth for another grind between the teeth – a process known as 'chewing the cud'. So, there is mechanical breakdown of the plant material by chewing and then chemical breakdown to even smaller components by the microbes. These sloshy smaller products are moved, by gut muscle contractions, through the third compartment, which is a conduit for appropriately sized food particles to pass into compartment number four.

This final compartment is often referred to as the 'true stomach' and is more akin to our own. From here digestion can continue in a more familiar way through the intestines until any waste is excreted as a humble cowpat. The significant fact to retain is that the nutrition from the cellulose has been made available not by the cow directly, but through a partnership with innumerable bacteria and other microorganisms that live in its gut.

Humans cannot subsist on grass alone because, simply, we don't have the microbes responsible for breaking down the cellulose, nor do we have a large stomach compartment available for them to live in happily. Eating chunks of our own lawn is unlikely to do us any real harm – though I would hardly recommend it – but it won't do us any good either: it'll simply come out the other end as undigested fibre.

Rabbits have a fascinating digestive system. They don't have a four-compartment stomach like cows and sheep, but they can still use cellulose as a source of nutrition. Instead, they are what are known as 'hind-gut fermenters', meaning the process of breaking down the cellulose in grass and other plants happens at the back end of their gut.

The plant material moves through the stomach and small intestine undigested, as would be the case for humans. Then, the rabbit's colon (part of the large intestine) separates the rougher, hard-to-digest fibre of the grass from the easy-to-digest fibre. Bear in mind this is all relative; for humans, none of this fibre is digestible due to its cellulose composition. The rougher fibre is passed as hard poo pellets, mainly during the day – the classic rabbit droppings we all recognise. The more digestible material then gets moved backwards into an area called the caecum, at the start of the large intestine. We all have a caecum, but ours is proportionately small; in a rabbit it can be ten times the size of its stomach. It is a large blind-ended sac full of microorganisms, and it's where much of the cellulose fermentation occurs in this species. Softer poo packets are then formed from the contents of the caecum and then passed. Yes, rabbits have two types of poo.

Now, you could be forgiven for thinking at this stage that the rabbit has just completely wasted its time; it spent hours getting the grass to a point where microbes have liberated its nutritional potential, only to pass it all straight out of its little bottom. But I'm afraid this is where you need to suspend your conventional beliefs about what constitutes appropriate table manners. These blackberry-like rabbit poops, the shining caecotrophs or 'night faeces', are then simply swallowed whole straight from under its cute little tail.

'Waste not, want not'; it is a very ingenious way of obtaining nutrition via a second pass through the front end of the digestive tract. It's not something you usually get to see as this activity is performed under the cloak of darkness in hutches or burrows, and it certainly isn't a feature of Beatrix Potter's Peter Rabbit books. However, it is a process that is important to understand as a vet who treats rabbits on a regular basis.

Changes in a rabbit's feeding habits, such as reduced appetite or not consuming night faeces, are good indications that something is awry. Rabbits, clearly, have a unique and very efficient gut system, but it needs to be fed with a regular supply of fibre. So, a rabbit that stops eating needs to be dealt with quickly or it may develop gut stasis. This is the cessation of movement through a rabbit's gastrointestinal tract and is a very serious issue that could lead to death. If we encounter a rabbit with gut stasis, we will immediately give them subcutaneous fluid (an injection of fluid under the skin which will disperse around the body) to keep them hydrated, a motility drug to stimulate gut movement, and, if they are not eating, a fibre-laden paste squirted directly into the mouth as an instant food.

Sometimes rabbit owners will bring in their rabbits believing they are suffering from diarrhoea, as they've found a dark, sticky mess in the fur around the rabbit's rear end. In fact, diarrhoea in rabbits is rare in my experience, and the mess is usually an accumulation of uneaten night faeces. The big question, then, is what has caused the lack of appetite for these nocturnal nuggets. Subsequently, we go on a hunt for the underlying issue, which can be varied and range from dental problems to an inappropriate diet.

On one occasion I recall being foxed. A friend brought in their rabbit with the complaint that it was 'not acting right, off food and not pooing'. Poppy was a sole rabbit allowed to roam freely in the garden. Had she eaten something she shouldn't have? I admitted her and gave the usual emergency treatment, then waited and monitored her, hoping that her guts would crank up their activity and return to normal. They did, but not before revealing the reason for her malaise. It appeared that a friendly wild rabbit which had been hanging about recently, Mr. McRabbit, as my friends called him, had been a little too friendly: Poppy had been pregnant with twins!

In the wide and extraordinarily varied world of veterinary medicine, you can't possibly know it all, let alone predict every possible outcome. We have what are called our 'core competencies', the set of vital skills a student must have before they can graduate with a veterinary degree. After that, of course, we gather experience, but additionally we are obliged to keep up to date with developments in knowledge and techniques by participating in continuing professional development – CPD.

Where needed, we can often check or refresh information 'on the hoof'. For a lot of the more unusual or challenging cases, there will always be some referencing and researching that goes on. We will frequently discuss cases among ourselves – within the team, and, when stumped, with enlisted specialist help. The latter is so much easier in these days where digital X-rays, photos and clinical notes can be sent instantly by email to anywhere in the world. And of course, with each case, you beef up the knowledge base in your brain.

It matters not that we are located in a remote corner of the country; every vet here takes their professional development very seriously. You're never too old to learn – if you think you are, it may be time to retire! We learn from attending courses – always useful if there's a practical element. We learn from online webinars – so much is now done this way, forced on everyone by the coronavirus pandemic. We learn from books, journals, web resources, pharmaceutical companies offering new medicines, and, of course, from each other. All of this helps us improve both our confidence and our skills, and even refreshes the basics on animals we might think we already know, quite literally, inside out.

A few years ago now, I went to a CPD conference and attended a lecture on rabbits. A lot of it was just a useful reminder of things I had learnt a long time ago, but as always, I acquired a few gems of wisdom that were totally new to me. One of those was on the topic of diagnosing the difference between a gut blockage (an intestinal obstruction) and a case of gut stasis. In both circumstances the rabbit will have stopped defecating, but their treatments are very different: a blockage requires surgery, whereas stasis can be treated medically, as outlined earlier. Unless the belly was noticeably beginning to bloat, I always found it pretty tricky to diagnose a blockage purely from a physical examination, but the lecturer gave me some vital new information.

As if to justify the value of CPD, within weeks of this conference I was presented with a rabbit displaying exactly this issue. It had stopped pooing and did have a bit of a swollen abdomen, but I couldn't be sure it definitely had a blockage. The wisdom I gained from the lecture, quite bizarrely to my mind, was that a blockage could be confirmed or dismissed by checking the rabbit's blood-sugar level.

A rabbit's blood sugar will rise with disease and stress, but the lecturer had informed us that if it goes above a certain threshold, it will almost certainly be due to a blockage. I honestly can't tell you why an elevated blood-sugar level indicates a blockage, but sure enough, I took this rabbit's blood-sugar level and was left in no doubt that surgery was required.

That afternoon, with the rabbit under anaesthetic, I opened it up and found a small dark bulge in its small intestine. It was a 'trichobezoar', which is the very fancy scientific name for a hairball (you are very welcome to memorise that term to wow your friends with, perhaps when someone's cat vomits a trichobezoar onto a carpet!). Rabbits, like cats, inevitably take in hair when grooming. What happens on occasion is that a little bundle of this can cause an obstruction. Unfortunately, surgically cutting into rabbit intestine to remove the blockage presents a very real practical problem. The small intestine is incredibly narrow – so narrow, in fact, that we are unable to stitch it without causing obstruction ourselves. What do we do then? How do we get the hairball out? Again, the rabbit lecture had offered the solution.

In all my time in practice I had neither diagnosed a rabbit's gut blockage through a blood-sugar reading nor conducted the procedure that I was about to perform on this rabbit, but the lecture loaned me the confidence to attempt both. Essentially, I 'milked' or massaged the rabbit's small intestine to work the trichobezoar along within it. Ever so gently, I squeezed this tiny dark hairball all the way along the tube until it headed out into the wide-open sea: the rabbit's large intestine.

It's surprising what can bring joy to a vet. A pile of poo at the rear of a previously blocked animal is definitely worthy of a fist pump. When the rabbit came round from its anaesthetic and passed faeces, I was immensely pleased with myself. The owner, too, was so appreciative that I indulged myself in a small moment of heroism. The bunny made a full recovery and I haven't needed to milk a rabbit intestine since, but it underscored the value of never resting on your laurels and continuing to push yourself to learn at every available opportunity.

Almost imperceptibly, the day length began to increase. As we progressed towards the end of winter, there was a spell of slightly milder weather. It suddenly felt warmer and lighter, a firm indication the cold season really was drawing to its close. Despite the fact the pleasant patch was followed up by another spell of dreich days, it felt like spring was finally emerging from a box that it wasn't going to be so easily forced back into.

A scattering of snowdrops and then daffodils emerged in Thurso's parks and gardens and gradually we became aware that our rural workload was increasing. Spring brings a palpable feeling of new hope and positivity to the northern Highlands, but there is a subtle change in our psychology too. Every single staff member at D. S. McGregor & Partners knows only too well what is coming up next.

The busiest season of our year brings mixed feelings with it. On one hand, there is a nervous energy and an excitement. No matter how many lambing and calving seasons you've endured, there is always that thrill that bubbles up as it gets going; bringing new life into the world never grows dull. On the other hand, you also know that the start of spring means the end to your chance of ever feeling fully rested until several months have passed. It is a truly disruptive period, with frantic shifts on call and lots of time away from your bed and your family.

I could easily have not taken a job in a rural practice like our one in Thurso, but I wouldn't want it any other way. As tough as spring can be, it is also the most exciting, interesting and rewarding of our seasons. Get through it all and we later receive the deep satisfaction of seeing the fruits of our labour grazing and growing in the fields as we pass by on our rounds.

The truth is, in life and work, if you want to get a real sense of achievement, then it's unlikely to come easily. The best rewards are often found through hard graft and by persevering in challenging situations. And therein lies a recipe for some of the best stories …

Spring

Chapter Seven

A Handcrafted Bumhole

Springtime in the countryside. It loans itself to picture-perfect images of snow-white lambs frolicking in the fields behind their mums. Innocence, beauty, freshness and a certain wholesome simplicity. Unfortunately, the gritty reality may not reflect these qualities down on the farm or in our surgery's large-animal wing. The patient that has just arrived is definitely a case in point.

'Well, I just seen him wagging his tail, he was trying to pass dung but ...' Farmer David's eyes drift down to the Texel lamb trotting gingerly around the surgery car park. 'He seemed to be struggling. There was something odd about him' – he lets out a self-conscious chuckle – 'so, I investigated.'

What David discovered was ... his five-hour-old lamb had been born without an anus.

It's now late March and the lambing and calving season is under-way. Naturally, you'd imagine the mainstay of our farm work to revolve around the safe delivery of lambs or calves that have found themselves in tricky positions within their mothers. That is largely true, but once those newborns are out and breathing the fresh air, they present with their own diseases and disorders. Believe it or not, the extraordinary-seeming abnormality found in this Texel lamb may be presented to us for surgical correction a handful of times every season.

Indeed, due to the huge number of sheep we serve, even a rare condition like having no bum will occur relatively often, but many such lambs might never receive surgery. It needs to be understood that farmers will make a decision to treat their animals based on very different criteria than those used by pet owners. The treatment of farm animals is driven more by economics than emotion. For any condition, the cost of treatment will be weighed against the value of the animal and the chance of that animal recovering from the treatment. A farmer will only stay in business if the ultimate value of the animal at market or as a future breeder is greater than other costs involved in rearing it to that point, and these will include medication and vet fees.

So, are animals left to suffer en masse? No, of course not; the opt-out for a 'no treatment' situation is euthanasia. When done humanely, putting an animal to sleep is unarguably the ultimate in the relief of suffering. Euthanasia is a welfare-conscious alternative. It may sound cold, callous and unemotional to those readers coming from a less rural background, but profits and margins are not normally considerations for pet owners – although it cannot be said that cost never enters the equation even for them.

It is not that farmers don't care about their animals – quite the contrary. Providing good care and sentimental attachment are not inseparable concepts. Livestock keepers take great pride in looking after their charges, in creating fine, healthy specimens; and they love to see them thriving and looking well. Of course, an unavoidable spin-off to this is that the end product is likely to be of better quality and higher value, whether that refers to a breeding animal that will take up residence in a flock or herd, or the meat on a consumer's plate. Everyone's a winner.

Yet, to paint it so black and white is to oversimplify things. I regularly come across farmers who'll let sentiment get the better of them and ask for a potentially uneconomic procedure to be performed because they just feel it's the right thing to do for that animal. They'll even have favourites among their flocks and herds, and if, say, a cow has been faithfully productive for years, they'll turn a blind eye to the cost in order to give her a chance. Despite their often gruff and pragmatic reputation, many farmers have soft spots hidden on the inside, and the weathered, calloused skin from toiling in the elements isn't always as thick as it appears.

David's lamb might not have its anus, but it is in fine health in every other aspect of its physical make-up. In the womb of any species, the development of the embryo and then the foetus is a pretty complex affair, and I think we'll all agree it's just downright amazing when we think about it. From the bundle of jack-of-all-trade cells formed soon after fertilisation, different cells take on specific roles to spawn the various tissues and organs that make up a body. The coordination of how this occurs – how each tissue subsequently takes up its place and joins up and interrelates with others – is mind-boggling and still not fully understood. It's surprising that things don't go wrong more often.

We are all familiar with what a back passage and a bum are. To be technical: the rectum, as we all know, makes its exit into the world through the skin at a muscle-regulated opening called the anus. During the development of this lamb, the anus never formed and the rectum didn't join up to it. Rather than a tube opening to the world through the anus, the rectum came to a blind end in the pelvis; close to it, but not linked up, was a hole-less bit of skin where the anus should have been. It was as if two teams had been asked to build a tunnel through a mountain. Team A were creating the tunnel (the rectum) and team B were tasked with simultaneously cutting out an exit arch and installing barriers (the anus). The two would ultimately meet and join their projects together to complete the job. However, team B decided to take the money and run, leaving the tunnel without an exit strategy.

The scientific name for this is 'atresia ani'. The lamb would be unaware of any problem initially and would suckle its mother, but soon, with nothing voiding at the back end, it would start to feel very full and, without surgery, ultimately die.

At least David was sharp in spotting his lamb's deficiency. It sounds like something anyone should easily be able to spot: a lamb without its anus; but you have to bear in mind that during lambing season farmers will have many newborn lambs to care for, and deliver, right across their sheds or fields. It can be a manic time, and something small and discreet missing from underneath a lamb's tail really isn't that obvious. Lambs are frequently born as part of twins or triplets too, so you can imagine how a farmer might look into a pen, see all the newborns suckling from their mum as normal, plus notice faeces left by the lamb's entirely healthy siblings, and then make the reasonable assumption that everything was fine with every animal.

Fortunately, in the grand scheme of things that can go wrong in foetal development, not having an anus sits very much in the shallow end of the pool. Because the rectum is there under the skin in David's lamb, if I can make a bumhole in the skin, open up the rectum and stitch the two together – doing what nature failed to do – then there's a chance I can save this animal.

Some really quite gory cases of other developmental mishaps sadly do crop up on very rare occasions. We see lambs and calves born with two heads, or with five legs. 'Water belly' can also occur, where fluid retention occurs in a big pot-bellied abdomen, but the rest of the baby animal is fine. We have what I've heard called 'teddy bear lambs', where fluid has gathered throughout the body and under the skin of the foetus, producing an extremely bloated and ballooned animal; these, and water bellies, may live for a few minutes after delivery before they inevitably pass away. Sometimes a foetus can even be inside out, with internal organs developing outside of its body.

As well as extra bits, it can happen that parts of the body will fail to develop; just a vestige or ghostly suggestion of what should have been there exists. As well as the anus, this can happen with an entire segment of bowel. If the final few inches of bowel are missing, then the blind end of the rectum is non-existent and so is not sitting in position just under the skin; thus, it is impossible for a surgeon to find it for 'new bum creation'. From the outside all you see is no bumhole, so these cases look identical to animals with simple atresia ani, but for them there is no hope of us fixing them.

With David's lamb, this is the big differentiation I want to make: is this a case of 'simple' atresia ani or a futile case where there is no bowel awaiting me on surgical exploration? If the latter, I would have to advise euthanasia. You can get a hint that a rectum awaits you on surgery by putting a little bit of pressure on the lamb's abdomen and then gently feeling the area under the tail where the anus should be. If you detect a tiny bulge coming out towards the skin, that is a strong indication that the lamb's bowel is fully formed and what you are feeling is the blind ending of the rectum, which is filled with faeces. Theoretically then, all you need to do is cut a hole in the skin where the anus should be, find the rectum, relieve all the pressure, and stitch it open. Easier said than done!

It may sound pretty straightforward, but having to form a handcrafted bum is a very messy, very finicky and delicate feat of surgery. If you were to simply hack in there, just to alleviate the lamb of its uncomfortable load as quickly as possible, you could easily end up losing the minute edges of the thin rectum as all the backed-up faeces explodes out of the animal's rear. You must hang on to those rectal edges if you are to successfully stitch them to the outer skin and complete the bespoke bottom.

Farmer David looks on nervously from the doorway of our lambing shed. I can sense his concern as I squeeze the tummy of his little Texel lamb, but I am quietly optimistic. I can feel a subtle pouch under the skin, so my instinct is telling me this is far more likely to be atresia ani than a case where a significant length of this lamb's bowel is missing. I've accosted vet Margaret to be my assistant, and she's pulled on her waterproofs to hold the lamb still while I operate.

In the last chapter I mentioned that risk is always associated with anaesthesia. The last thing we want to do is fully anaesthetise an animal that's only a few hours old unless we have no alternative. For atresia ani in lambs, I mitigate any danger by opting to keep the lamb awake and administering local anaesthetic instead. I reach for a brown glass bottle filled with the local. With Margaret bracing the lamb on a towel covering the operating table, I use a small needle and syringe to inject the anaesthetic into the lamb's rear, effectively numbing the surgical area without the lamb needing to lose consciousness at all.

There is a helpful sign indicating where I should start the procedure on the lamb's skin itself. 'Ah yes, there's a little mark on the skin there,' I note, as I rub my middle finger on what seems little more than a tiny spot. It is 'essence of bum', a ghostly mark where nature thought about making a bum but decided not to, for whatever reason. Extending my mountain tunnel imagery, it seems someone had marked 'Start here' on the mountainside for team B before they absconded. Now I know where I need to head, and I cut a hole in the skin at that point with my scalpel blade.

You might think that, given the lamb's rectum is likely to be bulging with poo, it would then be easy to locate the blind end of this tube. However, I'm working in a small space, and other bits of tissue, as well as the bleeding from my incision, are obscuring my view. One thing you learn very quickly in your career as a surgeon is that things in real life – when under the knife – rarely appear as distinct as they do on the pages of an anatomy textbook.

Margaret places a little pressure on the abdomen again, and I notice the slight swelling coming towards me through the lamb's pelvic canal. 'That's it. I'm pretty sure.' I feel in the gap with the tip of my little finger, gently prodding at the bulge. 'I hope there's faeces in here.' I grip the tissue with my tweezers and carefully snip into it with a pair of surgical scissors. 'There we are!' I've struck oil. All of a sudden, a triumphant beer-coloured liquid shoots out of the new bum-in-progress, as if someone had just opened a pressurised sewer. Fortunately, this first poo doesn't smell!

All newborn mammals pass their first faeces – called meconium – soon after birth. It might be reasonable to ask where this has come from if the young one has not yet suckled its mother. It is formed because the foetus takes in material as it drinks the fluid it is floating in within the womb. Like brown tar, meconium is normally very sticky and, believe me, doesn't wash off your waterproofs as easily as the more abundant and familiar adult poo. I'm sure there must be a market for meconium as a new DIY product to seal baths and showers. This lamb, oddly, had a huge amount of clear mucus fluid in addition to the tarry meconium, all desperate to fire out of the hole once I'd made it. The small things in life can bring so much pleasure; once again, I find myself elated at the sight of a large pile of poo. However, the fiddly work is about to begin.

With the lamb relieved of what turned out to be a quite considerable burden, I begin the process of handcrafting the bumhole. I take the edges of the now-open end of the rectum and start the precision work of stitching it to the edge of the hole I cut through the skin of the lamb's rear. They would not be easy stitches even in the best of conditions. The area I'm working in is tiny, and so must be the stitches. I've borrowed the eye kit from the small-animal wing, with its finer instruments. I suture (stitch) in all directions: in terms of a clock face, I lay stitches at twelve, three, six and nine o'clock initially and then fill in the gaps until I have formed a new cuff at the end of the sleeve of rectum.

Delaying me constantly in my pursuit is the surprising amount of faecal matter that continues to dribble across my surgical site, onto the table and down onto the floor. 'I wasn't expecting that much to come out,' Margaret comments. At one point I use my arm to sweep the soggy layer of goo on the operating table onto the floor in order to clear my workspace.

'It would be easier if you did just stop pooing now,' I chuckle as I try to place the final diminutive stitch. Then, at last, bum complete. Where nature had failed on this occasion, I am pleased to have lent her a hand.

It was a dirty task which might turn your stomach as a reader; but put your sensibilities to one side and, honestly, just imagine how awful it must be for the animals born with such a small but significant defect. I'm sure all of us have experienced the discomfort of constipation at some point in our lives, but to be physically unable to go *at all* would be a pretty unpleasant way to die, especially when you'd not yet had an opportunity to enjoy living.

If you haven't been completely put off by the slightly grim content in this story, you might be wondering how this lamb will regulate his bowel movements going forward. I haven't connected any muscles or nerves during my surgery, so the answer is: this lamb will never have any voluntary control over its bowel movements. But it is fair to ask, does this matter? A sheep is functionally incontinent anyway; they pretty much unthinkingly go as they please, whenever the moment takes them. I wouldn't be surprised to discover that someone has house-trained a sheep, but, as a rule, we never ask them to use voluntary bowel control. All that matters is that this newborn lamb has a chance at life, and the opportunity to grow up while comfortably executing one of the most basic bodily functions, in the fields, alongside the rest of his flock.

Margaret scoops the lamb off the table and holds it under her arm. It bleats and nuzzles her waterproof top, looking for Mum and her milk: reassuring signs that all has gone well. She passes him back to a relieved-looking farmer David. 'Keep checking him,' I advise. 'Within 24 hours he should have faeces coming out the other end.' By this I mean faeces of a character that has been formed from milk the lamb has suckled, distinct from meconium. David thanks us and places the lamb into the boot of his car, and I get down to the task of sloshing and squeegeeing all the poo from the lambing shed's surgical area down into the drains. *Hopefully that little lad will be okay now,* I think to myself.

Twelve days later, just a couple of miles south of the most northerly point on mainland Britain, the television crew catches up with David on his windswept farm. 'Oh, he's fine,' he laughs, as the lamb with the fine-tailored anus skips along happily behind his mother. 'Guy's done a good job. It was worth taking the chance.'

Chapter Eight

Birthing Problems and How to Solve Them

Up here in Caithness and what I shall refer to as 'north Sutherland', farming is central to life. If you are not directly involved in farming yourself, you will certainly know someone who is. In Scotland there are more sheep than people, and almost one-third of the UK's entire breeding beef cattle herd reside here as well. According to the Scottish National Farmers Union, 80 per cent of Scottish land is under agricultural use, and in rural Scotland, agriculture is the third-largest employer. Scottish lamb and beef producers are known worldwide for yielding some of the highest-quality meat and maintaining the best welfare standards. Farming, it is fair to say, is a very big deal in this country, and has long been a massive part of the culture of our northerly region.

In the book *Caithness Archaeology: Aspects of Prehistory*, authors Andrew Heald and John Barber present evidence that suggests formal farming was introduced here as far back as the Neolithic period, around 4000 BC. Archaeologists have excavated remains that also indicate those early residents of Caithness kept pigs and cattle, as well as growing wheat and barley. Back then, with slightly elevated temperatures, they reckon the Flow Country was considerably less boggy; but this county's lower altitude and profile soon lent itself to the development of rolling pastureland, and latterly, wide-scale commercial farming.

In the land around our practice there are some 700 farms, ranging from the largest, at over 1,000 acres, right down to the 'crofts' (traditional smallholdings of 50 acres or less). There is only a little dairy milk production hanging on in the county, and there are a few pigs and goats and some novelty species such as alpacas – and even ostriches in years past – but the overwhelming majority of farming revolves around cows and sheep for the production of beef and lamb. The cattle are generally kept in what are termed 'suckler herds', where the calves are born on the farms and suckle their mothers until they are usually between 7 and 10 months old, before being sold off as 'stores' for someone else to fatten up for meat production.

Sheep are seasonal breeders, giving birth in the spring, but cows can give birth at any time of year. We see a few batches of calves born in the autumn, but the majority of farmers want to make use of the abundance of fresh grass available during the warmest months. That means aiming for most of the calves to be born in the spring too. So, thousands of sheep and cows, right across these northern counties, are all giving birth during the same intense period every single spring.

Most births will happen naturally without complication, or with a little help from the farmers themselves. Someone once asked me if we attended every birth on the farms that we serve.

Thankfully not! We would have to employ dozens more vets on a temporary basis each spring if that were the case. We just get called for the tricky ones. In fact, these represent quite a small proportion of all births; but, with so many animals in labour, it doesn't take too many emergencies to see us worked off our feet, right around the clock.

The biggest beef and sheep farms in the world, in places like America, China and Australia, can have thousands of animals on land comfortably in excess of 100,000 acres. Farming on such an intensive industrial scale means the individual farm can afford to build everything to high specification for whatever task the farmers need to perform – from shearing, to gathering, to giving the animals their inoculations – and will happily invest huge sums in the technology to mechanise and streamline as much of its production line as possible. Places like that may even opt to employ an on-farm vet who is available 24/7 to look after any health problems they encounter with their animals.

Farming on that scale in our patch of Scotland would require someone to monopolise almost every farm and merge them into a single monstrous enterprise. I am happy that is unlikely to ever be the case. Where multiple small-to-medium farms exist, either the vets have to travel from farm to farm to see animals in person or the farmers themselves have to bring them into the surgery, in our case to our lambing shed.

There are practical limitations to which animals we can see in the lambing shed. Well-behaved horses could be, and often are, treated in our large-animal wing; but, although a full-size cow might fit in the room, it would be unmanageable without proper handling facilities, so we tend to see most cows and bulls in situ, on the farm. When it comes to smaller farm animals such as calves and sheep, if the farmer can bring them to us it makes much more sense both economically (no call-out charge for the farmer) and for our own time efficiency. We can comfortably get through several lambings or cases of sick calves or lambs in the time it takes to get to a single distant farm call. Having that one-stop shop makes the sheer volume of cases more manageable from our side, but it also gives us a bespoke-built clinical environment that contains every-thing we need for the majority of the season's likely procedures, and a good few unexpected ones too.

When it comes to the care and treatment of animals, we might draw a rough analogy: in some respects, an animal owner could be seen to be in a similar position to that of a parent with their own child. The parent is charged with caring for their children, and they can give simple medications, a bit of Calpol perhaps or a plaster to cover a wounded knee. They are also the ones who will raise the alarm if there is something seriously medi-cally wrong with their child. They will call the doctor, alert the paramedic, or take them directly to the hospital themselves; but at no stage would a parent strap their child to the kitchen table and attempt to operate on them with the family cutlery, nor ply them with medicines they weren't trained in using. Apart from common sense, there are issues of legality. This would be very much the case for pet owners, horse clients and farmers with respect to their charges.

Rural vets inhabit an important niche and play a valuable role in a farmer's business. I would like to think that most farmers appreciate the specialised knowledge and skill set brought by the veterinary profession in relation to the care and performance of their livestock. Moreover, there are certain tasks that only we, as trained professionals, can perform on animals – this is enshrined in law in the Veterinary Surgeons Act. Prescription medicines can only be prescribed by a qualified vet and practically every surgical procedure can only be undertaken by a vet too. Although, there are some deregulated procedures; for example, a farmer could dehorn or castrate an animal under certain conditions.

When it comes to the spring season, a farmer may well be capable of delivering a calf or lamb that has found itself in a tricky position inside its mum, but if it's anything more troublesome, then that's where we step in. If the call comes through to me, I might just ask a few questions to establish a little more about the 'dystocia' – a medical word meaning a problematic labour – just so I have an idea of what I might expect on arrival. Before we dive into what exactly the problem could be, let's first look at how the normal birth process – or to give its technical name, 'parturition' – occurs. The physical process is very similar in all mammals, including humans. There are variations from species to species at a cellular and chemical level, much of which is still not completely understood, but here is what we know about cows and sheep.

In its simplest terms, labour is associated with an increase in foetal cortisol as the foetus approaches its time to make an appearance. Cortisol is a steroid hormone we all release under stress, but it's best not to think of this as a stressed foetus banging on the womb in a panic, crying, 'Let me out!' (although it is a useful bit of cartoon imagery to help our brains get a handle on it). The cortisol circulates into the placenta and mother's body, initiating a cascade of biochemical events and hormonal changes. Indeed, we can induce labour in cows by injecting cortisol-type drugs.

The cervix is the cylinder-shaped neck and exit portal of the uterus (the womb), and up until now it has been tightly closed to keep the calf, placenta and fluids contained. Hormonal changes encourage it to dilate. The womb's muscle also starts to contract, squeezing the uterine contents – including the calf – towards the opening cervix. The pressure on the cervix creates a self-reinforcing cycle known as the Ferguson reflex, whereby more hormones are released and feed back into the process. Once the foetus has been pushed far enough into the birth canal (comprising the cervix and vagina), the mother feels the urge to push with her abdominal muscles. This combination of dilation, slippy fluids and the contraction of womb and abdominal muscles works to usher the foetus into the world, whereupon it becomes a 'neonate' – a newborn.

During the first stage of labour, it is more a case of things going on inside. The mother is feeling a bit weird and knows something is most definitely up. In sheep or cows, you might notice they seclude themselves from the rest of the flock or herd as the mum's cervix is just starting to open. A water bag – the fluid-filled sac from the placenta – will appear visibly at the back end (her vulva). The second stage of labour is the abdominal pushing phase that helps the foetus out, and the third stage is the delivery of the after-birth: the placenta.

Going back to our call from the farmer then, when someone has called us with a sheep or cow experiencing some form of dystocia – a birth that has got stuck at some point during stages one or two – the information they provide might allow us to determine whether we are dealing with a foetal problem or a maternal problem.

A classic maternal problem encountered mainly in sheep and from time to time in cows is 'ringwomb'. That's when the mother's cervix hasn't opened as it ordinarily should. For some reason, the aforementioned cascade has frozen like computer software at a critical moment. What's worth remembering as a vet, though, is that there is *true* ringwomb, and there's just impatience! True ringwomb is when, no matter how long you wait or what you try, the cervix will simply never open up. In that instance, I know I'll be conducting a caesarean section. Often, more time is all that is needed, and occasionally certain medications may help. Understandably, farmers become anxious; they don't want to lose the lambs or calf by leaving it all too long. So, I must treat the human rather than the sheep with a draught of reassurance and a dose of patience. It will often naturally take just a little longer for the cervix to fully open, particularly if it's the ewe's first labour. Some of these cases return hours later and require surgery, but others we don't hear from again, nature having taken its course.

On the other side of dystocia are the foetal problems. These are typically 'malpresentations', the word we use to describe how a lamb or a calf has ended up lying in an unusual position inside its mum, which stops them from being born without aid. So, what is a 'normal' or standard presentation? The most common is known as 'anterior presentation', where both forelegs of the lamb or calf stretch out through its mother's birth canal in a diving position, with its head resting between them, forming a triangular shape between the nose and the two front hooves. The other normal presentation is 'posterior presentation', with the lamb or calf coming out backwards, back legs outstretched, hooves appearing first.

Before we go any further, it must be said that dystocia can occur even with a normal presentation and an open cervix, simply because the calf or lamb is too big for the hole it's intended to pass through. This is a relative phenomenon and will come about due to either foetal oversize or maternal undersize. A mother with a narrow pelvis is a risk factor for dystocia, and it is now possible to do pelvic measuring in cows so that particularly narrow ones can be weeded from the breeding herd. Even in a roomy pelvis, a whopper of a calf or lamb is always going to present problems. The sticking points in the foetus are usually wide shoulders, a deep keel on the chest or a big back end (wide hips).

Frequently, all that is needed to help the lamb or calf through the birth canal is traction – a pull to augment the push occurring from the inside. However, even the pull of one person can be too much for lambs; if a lamb cannot be delivered by the strength of one person, then you shouldn't be pulling it! Cows and calves, on the other hand, can take more tension. A calving jack can be attached to the calf's legs by ropes. This jack is a ratchet on a shaft that directs the pull exerted on the calf back onto the cow's rear end (in the same way that, when pulling out a stubborn root in the garden, you direct the pull back to the ground through your boots). Such calving aids must be used with sense and sensitivity; they allow one person to pull with the power of several.

Back to how lambs and calves can be presented at birth. Let's talk about calves, but most of the following applies to lambs too.

Anterior presentation is the ideal. It is possible to assess with our hands the room available for the calf's chest and shoulders, but there is a certain amount of faith that the back end of the calf will slide out nicely; it is practically impossible to reach in to feel the calf's hips, and cases of 'hip lock' will occur, which you develop knacks to cope with. Posterior presentation is fairly common and will usually see a normal healthy delivery too, but there are some additional risks. This time you can feel the size of the calf's back end but struggle to assess the chest and shoulders.

A calf's chest is roughly cone-shaped, narrow at the head end and wide at the back where it meets the abdomen. The ribcage is quite springy, so when the calf is diving out head first it is naturally compressed then springs open again after delivery. In posterior presentation, the wide edges of the cone – the back of the calf's ribcage – engage with the mother's pelvis first, and the bigger the chest, the bigger the chance of the ribs catching and breaking under the pressure. It is possible to reduce the risk of the ribs catching by pulling the calf out horizontally or even with the hind legs pointing slightly upwards, as opposed to the more usual tendency to deliver diagonally downward towards the ground, as would be the case for an anterior calf. If a few ribs go pop, they will heal, but in severe cases the newborn unfortunately won't make it. So, a large posterior calf may trigger a Caesar more readily than a large anterior calf, to be on the safe side.

The most common malpresentations include 'leg back', where the calf is in the anterior position but with one foreleg tucked back under itself inside its mother, and the other facing forward out of the birth canal alongside its own head. Of course, both forelegs might be tucked back and so just the head is facing out. In both situations we will occasionally create some slack by pushing the calf slightly back into its mother, then squeeze a hand through into the uterus and manipulate the backward-facing leg forward. With calves, we use hands and arms for these manipulations, with lambs, often just fingers. The pressure on a calf's neck when just its head alone is wedged in the birth canal is such that the whole head and tongue can swell alarmingly. They can look bizarrely malproportioned once delivered and may need to receive their first feed by stomach tube as the huge tongue prevents suckling. It's amazing how they settle down, though.

Another common finding after sliding your arm into the back end of a cow is a calf in 'head back' position. Here the forelimbs are forward in their correct anterior positions, but the calf's head is facing away from the opening and looking back into the cow, towards its own back leg. To fish out the head, we may push the legs back into the uterus too. That may sound counterproductive, but it creates space to work. Tagging the legs with ropes can be a prudent move to aid in their retrieval once the head has been redirected, then you can deliver the calf as normal.

More fun malpresentations include the 'breech'. This is where I find the layperson has looser terminology than that which we would use. A true breech is not coming backwards in the same way as a posterior presentation. Rather, it presents with no feet; it is coming bum and tail first. Both its hind legs are tucked under its body and pointing in the direction of its own head, like a high diver in pike position. Occasionally some have their hind legs bent as if kneeling – these are much easier to reposition. Delivering a breech can be a challenge, especially in a long-legged calf where you have to work with the tips of your fingers to gain the reach. I slip my hand into the womb and try to get my finger into the crook of the calf's hock joint. I then work away at it to bend it, thus bringing the hoof within reach. Then, in a bike-pedalling motion, I pop the foot out into the birth canal, being careful to protect the uterus from the points of the hock and hoof as they move; it is not impossible to perforate the uterus if too much force is used. It is a two-arm job in a cow, but in a ewe, where everything is scaled down, it requires a very clever use of one hand as if it were two. Then I do it all over again with the second hind leg, but this is often harder now that the first leg is in my way. Once the legs are retrieved, we effectively have a posterior presentation and hopefully deliver the calf uneventfully, and I have to say, delivering a breech is a very satisfying experience.

'Upside down' is another malpresentation. It means, instead of the calf's spine facing up and adjacent to its mum's spine, its spine is facing down towards its mum's udder, so the calf is effectively belly-up. They are usually stuck pretty fast in that position, and turning them can be a bit of a nightmare. If the calf is a good size, then they can end up as Caesars. Some are not fully belly-up but are falling to one side and can be more amenable to one of the following techniques. I might try repelling the calf into the womb a little to where there's a bit more space to move, then have a direct attempt at turning the calf over with rotational force. If this fails, as it often will, my other technique is what I shall call my 'dynamic delivery'. I loop ropes onto the calf's legs and attach them to a calving jack. With the farmer using the jack under my strict instruction, I put both hands in the birth canal to try to rotate the calf. Where rotate *then* pull has failed, sometimes the simultaneous actions of rotate *and* pull will work to corkscrew the calf out.

Having covered the upside-down malpresentation, it makes sense to mention something here that, to the uninitiated, might appear superficially similar. A 'twisted womb' is the situation where the calf may well present in the upside-down position, but only for the simple reason that the whole uterus is upside down. To picture this condition, think of the uterus as being like a balloon filled with water, with the calf inside. Imagine you are holding the neck of that balloon, which represents the cervix. Now twist the balloon around. A twist of just 180 degrees would significantly narrow the opening at the neck of that balloon, but twist it 360 degrees and it will be completely closed. Of course, a full twist of 360 degrees may not leave the calf lying upside down, but getting it out is going to be troublesome.

When we find this condition in a ewe, there usually isn't the space to get hands in to fix the problem, so we'll tend to opt for a caesarean section. In a cow, however, we stand a chance of untwisting the womb, though many end up as Caesars too. We can often squeeze our hand through the neck of the 'balloon', feeling a tight spiral effect as we do so. It is, in theory, possible to know the direction of the rotation by feeling the spiral in the cervix, and so we know which way to twist it back. Next, we locate the most substantial bit of calf we can reach and start to push on it to effect the unwinding. Not as easy as it sounds! It is all done at arm's length with room for only one arm. The weight of the calf (50 to 70kg) plus the uterine fluid, with the huge cow's stomach pressed up against it, leaves me amazed that we do actually untwist many of them. Sometimes I resort to a rocking action, swinging the womb like a slow pendulum until it eventually flips over – like pushing a child's swing in the park higher and higher until it goes right over the top bar. I end up contorted, with my back against the cow's backside and my arm stuck out behind me into her back passage.

My shoulder often aches for days afterwards, but what a feeling of achievement when it falls into position and suddenly there is a wide-open canal to pull the calf through!

I remember once having two twisted womb cases during the same evening. I worked away at the first for 20 minutes before eventually getting that wonderful feeling of it rolling back into position so I could deliver the calf. The second cow, on a different farm, had an identical twist; what were the chances of that?! After my practice run earlier, I sorted the second twist in a jiffy. I then revelled in the stunned and thoroughly impressed expression on the farmer's face. 'I thought it was a certain Caesar,' he said.

A more involved technique for a twisted womb is, rather than untwist the womb itself, to untwist the cow. I have done this, but it is time-consuming and not always effective. The cow is cast (by that I mean made to lie down), then we effectively rotate her around her own womb by gripping her legs and quickly moving her from lying on one side to the other. This relies on the principle of inertia with respect to the womb – unless you try to improve your chances by flying in the face of health and safety and lying on the ground, hands in cow, trying to hold the calf in position as the mother revolves around it.

Mixed-up twins can present a whole range of fun and frustrating challenges. Putting your hand in to discover two heads or more than two feet means you're either dealing with a rare malformation or, more likely, a multiple birth where the youngsters are quarrelling over who gets to go first. To sort them out, I suggest you first choose a head or a leg and then simply don't let your fingers leave that calf until you have traced the other relevant parts attached to the same body. Sometimes tagging a leg with a rope can be useful so that once you've moved on to find the other, you can differentiate it again from the melee of body parts. Once you've managed to isolate the individuals, you then have to decide who is to be born first. It's not always obvious but I usually go for the animal that is closest to the opening, especially if it is in anterior presentation; it's likely to be the easiest, and removing that calf should give you much better access to the sibling lying in wait behind. Usually, the ease of delivery of the first calf gives you an indication of how easily the next will arrive, but then there's always the potential that its brother or sister might be a real lump, and so, rarely and frustratingly, a Caesar may still be needed at this stage.

Just to remind you, for the above dystocia conditions in calves, you can read 'lamb' too, as sheep encounter the same troubles.

I recall delivering a breech calf many years ago and the farmer, experienced as he was, asked me how I'd managed it. I paused with a cheeky smile on my face, and he responded, 'I see, why would you give away your trade secrets?' I don't feel I have given any trade secrets away in my ramblings in the previous few paragraphs. I could tell you until I'm blue in the face how to calve a cow or lamb a sheep, but you won't be able to do it until you actually do it. It is a very practical pursuit and experience counts for a lot. Tricky births are our bread and butter in the spring. If in doubt, call us out!

There is always a buzz in seeing lambs and calves splutter into this world, particularly if you've played an essential part in it all. For a vet, the more challenging the struggle, the more rewarding it can feel.

Chapter Nine

Twins in the Car Park

By the time April is underway we are well into the lambing and calving season, and it soon becomes a struggle to remember a time when we weren't all spending our on-call hours in the surgery's lambing shed, or down on a farm delivering lambs and calves. The rest of the practice's workload – the small-animal work, other routine farm work, the horse work – continues as normal alongside this huge heap of hard graft, but your body and mind soon adapt to it. Bright-tailed and bushy-eyed, we just carry on from job to job.

This spring the weeks have passed and, between us all, we soon saw almost the full spectrum of malpresentations and other impediments to normal birth. For the first season in a while, I haven't had to deal with a twisted womb. We did, however, find vet William being filmed dealing with a twisted womb in a ewe expecting triplets. We've seen and treated vaginal prolapses, torn uteruses and constipated lambs too, and the season has flowed forward with lots of happy deliveries, less sleep than we would like, and only a few moments of real sadness.

Sleep deprivation and repetition can soon see you sink into a slightly otherworldly autopilot setting, where you go from day to day without ever finding time to reflect on any of the wonderful outcomes of all your hard work. The *Highland Vet* cameras do help immortalise many moments, though, like when farmer Donald arrives in the practice car park with a Texel-cross ewe that's struggling to progress with her labour.

Donald is a very experienced stockman with over 60 years of farming under his belt. He's also a kindly man who cares greatly for his animals. I've worked with him many times over the years. If Donald senses there is any problem at all, he doesn't hesitate to pick up the phone and call the vets. Donald may be past the standard retirement age for most of society, but as with so many of the Caithness farmers, his passion for his work burns just as brightly as it ever did. Whenever he's on the subject of his animals, you can see in him the spark of a far younger man.

He opens the back of his trailer and peers in at his sheep through a pair of wire-frame spectacles. 'There's a problem somewhere, that's for sure,' he begins with concern. 'I don't think she's opening for lambing. There's something wrong.'

Donald's trailer has ample room for me to conduct the basic examination of the ewe, and indeed, unless we end up resorting to surgery, it's an ideal place for me to assist a normal vaginal delivery. For the comfort of the ewe it makes sense to not give her any additional stress by ushering her into the lambing shed, and indeed, selfishly I think, it would save me cleaning the whole place down afterwards too, which is always a bonus during this busiest of seasons.

We have had sheep turn up at our lambing shed in all sorts of vehicles over the years. There are strict legal requirements relating to the transport of farm animals, but concessions are granted for medical emergencies and veterinary treatment. Donald's trailer is perfect for transporting animals in both sickness and health, but we've had sheep arrive in everything from the back of a hatchback – where they can truly gunk up the upholstery of the family car in no time at all – right through to the boot of a Land Rover. The latter might sound very sensible, but actually lifting a heavy sheep to or from the waist-high rear platform is no mean feat, believe me. It could be a new event in the Highland Games alongside tossing the caber!

Grateful for the trailer, I pull on a pair of blue arm-length gloves as Donald fills me in on what he's discovered so far: 'I can't feel the lamb inside, so it must be far back.' I ease the ewe over onto her side. Donald has laid down a bed of fresh straw, and I call him in to restrain her at her front end.

Carefully, I slide my lubricated hand into the ewe's birth canal. 'Aye, she's tight,' calls Donald from the head. She is, it's true, but there are degrees of tightness that you come to recognise with experience. It feels like there is just enough room to attempt a delivery without putting the ewe or the lamb through unwarranted stress, but first I need to figure out quite why she hasn't already delivered naturally and uneventfully.

Introducing more of my arm, I can feel the lamb's legs and deduce it is in posterior presentation and upside down, which, as I mentioned in the previous chapter, means this lamb's spine is facing down towards the ewe's udder, with the lamb effectively belly-up. It just isn't going to get through the birth canal like that. To complicate things slightly, this ewe is also a 'gimmer', meaning she is a young, inexperienced ewe between her first and second shearing, and this is her very first pregnancy. Things are always likely to take a little longer with gimmers as they are much more prone to be tight. It's important I act quickly, but not hastily, to relieve the stress on her unborn young.

I ease the lamb towards the ewe's cervix, gripping the hind legs, before I apply firm but gentle force to rotate it into the correct position. I can't think of many other lines of work where such a critical process must be executed without the use of one of our major senses: sight. I don't know what goes on in the brains of other vets when they are lambing or calving, but I find I can 'see' what's going on inside the womb. Eyes aren't the only organ by which to see things. Bats and dolphins see using echoes of sound to form pictures in their brains; similarly, I find that the tactile input from the shapes and textures presented to my fingertips allows my mind's eye to form an image of the situation in the womb. All very useful when trying to work out how to solve problems of parturition.

As I work with Donald's ewe and lamb, I guess I first envisage the blank darkness of the ewe's birth canal, 'seeing' the open cervix as my hand enters it. I then feel the lamb's legs, the arrangements of joints telling me they are hind legs and that they are upside down. I add all this information to my picture of the lamb lying among the placenta and fluid. With trickier malpresentations, where legs and heads are coming at me from all directions, it can be difficult, and my brain must fill in the gaps between the snapshots my hand provides. In the end, if all goes to plan, I get to see the lamb for real, spluttering and shaking its head as it takes its first lung-opening breaths.

The birth canal is composed of soft tissue passing through the hard, bony pelvis. When the lamb or calf is filling practically the whole canal, it doesn't leave much room for your hand or arm to slide on past. With cows, as you insert your hand and start working to manipulate the infant, your presence will elicit the irrepressible urge for the mother to push hard with her abdominal muscles. I'm sure the cow has her own discomfort to think about, but it can also be genuinely physically painful for the vet. Bruises on our arms will occur from time to time, particularly after calvings. In sheep, being smaller, I find I'm left with sore finger joints more than bruises.

Until a Caesar is considered, assisting a birth is not about fancy equipment; yes, a calving jack is used for convenience, but a few strong bodies could substitute for that, as was the case in years gone by. It's all about using little more than the best instrument we have: ourselves. Muscles, tactile sense, dexterity – it's fundamentally a very physical event. Just man and beast, and perhaps some rope. Notwithstanding the skill that is also required, there is something about this part of a vet's work that still feels very down to earth and in touch with nature. It is probably one of the only things we do that the Highland farmers of Neolithic times would still be able to understand, recognise and identify with. Although I'm sure they would be fascinated by a metal calving jack.

'Right, I'll let you do the pushing, madam.' Having successfully rotated her lamb, I offer Donald's ewe a suggestion in the hope she might comply. Pushing out a lamb is always preferable to too much pulling. The lamb's back legs meet the fresh air first, followed by its rump, which I gently pull clear of her passage. Next, as a posterior presentation, the lamb's chest is about to encounter its mother's pelvis. Is it deep-chested? Will the wide back edge of the conical ribcage catch the pelvic brim and cause the ribs to pop one by one? Luckily, this lamb is pleasantly streamlined. *Phew.* With my right hand holding the back legs of the lamb together, and my left gripping on its upper thighs, this newborn slides out into the world. It is followed immediately by a great sploshing puddle of sticky brown-yellow fluid, and a very satisfied 'Great!' from Donald, who has been quietly crouching over the front end of his ewe.

It's a tup lamb – a strong and healthy boy. I wipe all the gunk from his face and mouth, even placing a finger inside to scoop out any residue, and he starts confidently inflating his lungs for the very first time. His eyes are wide and alert as I place him up by his mum's head. 'That's a good result,' I say to Donald.

'Aye,' he replies, 'magic!'

The variety in nature is what can make this job so fascinating at times. Some lambs are like this wee tup. They will pop out of their mums and immediately sit up, cough and splutter a little, and quickly get on with their lives, bright as a button. Others will come out not faring so well, and really struggling to breathe and lift their heads. Sometimes there is no obvious reason; other times it could just be the stress and pressure they've endured during a long or difficult birth, or they may be born a little prematurely with underdeveloped lungs.

Being born backwards, in posterior presentation, doesn't help either and can leave a lamb with a bit more fluid to clear before breathing becomes easy. The umbilical cord, attached to the lamb's belly, is its lifeline when in the womb. Without air to breathe, its oxygen supply comes through this 'hosepipe' from its mum's placenta. In humans this cord is often clamped and cut after delivery, but in animals, as a general rule, it breaks naturally. If being delivered head first, the youngster's head, and possibly its chest, might often be out in the air before the cord becomes squashed or taut enough to break. So, if the delivery is slow – perhaps the back end of the lamb gets stuck – then at least it will hopefully be able to start breathing, despite not quite being clear of its mother yet. Now flip this image and visualise a lamb arriving back legs first. The head is the last thing to reach open air and the cord will often have already broken by this point, thus oxygen supply is cut off. With the head still dunked in fluid inside the womb, the lamb will attempt to breathe. A speedy delivery is required or the worst can happen.

Breathing is the all-important focus once a lamb or calf has been delivered. In the first instance you'll clear the whole head, mouth and nostrils of any slimy fluid or obstruction. If no breaths are forthcoming, you then need to try something to stimulate breathing, fast. We have several tactics up our sleeves. Quite honestly, there are few things better for this than a piece of straw. It is inserted up the newborn's nose and wiggled about to stimulate a response. It's usually readily available to hand; Donald, for example, lined the floor of his trailer with it, and often you'll find a piece stuck in the fleece of the ewe anyway. Straw is just the right consistency to do the job: stiff enough to insert into the nose, but not so stiff that you're going to do any damage. Low-tech, but it works: the irritation will trigger a big sneeze or cough to blow out the gunge in the upper passages, and this is hopefully then followed by a deep breath.

If you sense there's fluid to be shifted from further down the airway or lungs, you might then suspend a newborn by its back legs, head to the ground, and use gravity to encourage the fluid to flow out to allow air in. For a calf this means hooking its waist up over a gate to hang it vertically. A hefty calf will take at least two folk and a little muscle and grunting to manage this – bear in mind its legs are still wet and slimy, so there's poor grip. Patting its chest as the calf hangs might help dislodge fluid within the lungs too. It's amazing how much clear gooey fluid can flow out on occasions. In lambs there is a more dramatic way to persuade fluid to move up and out of the airway: centrifugal force. The wee thing is taken by the back legs and then we spin ourselves at speed. Caution: make sure you have a good grip and that there are no obstacles in your radius!

With Donald's lamb already up on his feet by the ewe's head, I crouch down by her vulva. 'Let's see, there's an awful big thingy coming out here … Just the water bag.' The membrane-bound sac full of fluid that has been the lamb's home for the last few months has burst on its delivery. Now appearing is what I initially thought to be a residual pocket of this sac. However, in just the couple of minutes it has taken to get the newborn acquainted with his mum, the situation has developed somewhat back at the action end. This is not a ballooned portion of an old bag – it's a new one entirely!

The ewe is pushing naturally, so I grab the bag and burst it, slide my hand back into her birth canal and through into her uterus once again. There, I can feel a twin making its way towards me, feet and head first. I grip both its feet between thumb and middle finger and gently pull, and it is soon out on the straw. A little shake this time and its tiny pink tongue emerges from its mouth. Its dark eyes open. 'Auch!' exclaims Donald, chuckling to himself with glee, 'That's really great, Guy!'

Donald's eyes are alive with excitement as the first lamb stumbles around his mother's side, and I place the second on her fleece.

Even after all these years in the farming industry, and many hundreds of births, it's heart-warming to see he can still be thrilled by an event such as this successful delivery.

For farmers like Donald, retirement is not something they want to consider. Farming isn't just a job to them; it is a central part of who they are, it's a way of life. On farms that have a new generation coming through, the work naturally passes to the younger, less worn-out hands. But more often than not, you'll see the older farmer, well beyond retirement age, continue to put on his wellies and muck in every day. They'll have their wee jobs that they do, while the bulk of the heavier work is undertaken by those they have brought up and trained to take on their mantle. Stopping work altogether is not really an option, it's in their blood.

Even for those farmers who have no one to pass the farm on to, you'll find that many of them just steadily downsize, rather than giving up the work for good. Eventually, all they'll be left with is a puckle – a small handful – of animals, but they can't bring themselves to let all their livestock go. Take the animals away and you take away their reason for getting up in the morning. You take their identity. You take away their life.

Chapter Ten

The Highlands' Cows

It really would be a lot more convenient if lambing just abruptly finished one day in spring and calving started up the next. In reality, the sheep work may start to reduce as spring rolls on, but calving ramps up throughout, and so, in April and May, we are near-guaranteed to have to drag ourselves out of bed when taking our turn at on-call duties. Animals prefer to give birth in the still and calm of the night; we would prefer to be sleeping!

We do get a wee smattering of cow births in early February in Caithness, which is somehow still broadly classified as the start of our spring calving period. That always makes me chuckle. As if a northern Highland February, with all its wintry darkness and frozen edges, could ever be mistaken for spring! For the vast majority of the 30,000 head of cattle spread across Caithness and north Sutherland, you can expect them to be giving birth within the traditional spring window running from the beginning of March until the end of June. That serves to underline just how much the calving season dominates the calendar of our rural veterinary practice. Up here, the Thurso vets and those of our sister practice in Wick cover all calving emergencies for that huge herd that fall beyond the scope of farmhand assistance.

The practice has always had a general rule of 'no holidays at peak season'. They are outright prohibited in April and May; we need all hands to the pumps. Nights can roll seamlessly into days, with you conducting a Caesar on a farm in the twilight hours, before tending to an ailing dog first thing in the morning down at the surgery. It's always worth remembering that the farmers get absolutely no time off during this period either; at least we run our schedules to make sure our vets do get something of a break following a run on-call. Nonetheless, the season is physically and mentally exhausting when you're right in the thick of it.

Calving is a lot more physically demanding than lambing, by nature of the fact that the calf being delivered could weigh as much as the vet delivering it. Calving takes more time too: you have to drive to the farm, assess the cow, decide if it's a Caesar, operate, drive home, clean up your messy kit ready for the next one. Most lambings are generally dealt with more efficiently in the lambing shed at the practice.

It can really start to grind you down after a while. Often, the support staff will be loading up the vets with coffee and biscuits as they tumble in and out of the building. I don't think sleep deprivation is particularly good for anyone's health in the long term. There is a sense of just trying to hold on and get through until the light at the end of the tunnel appears as the peak is passed. That's not to say that the sense of deep reward just disappears into a cloud of extreme fatigue; the satisfaction of saving an animal in an acute emergency is always there. Plus, there is frequently room for a fair bit of fun along the way too.

A culture of good humour can run deep in workplaces where a degree of stress and fatigue comes as part of the job. There's really nothing quite like a jolly good laugh to alleviate some of the pressure.

April Fool's Day this year found us with new victims in the form of TV camera crew members. Vet William texted them all, saying there was a killer whale stranded on a beach needing urgent attention. Two of the crew rushed in and were poised ready, waiting at the surgery, beside themselves with excitement at the prospect of this amazing scoop. And then Amber, a crew member who had filmed the previous two series, breezed past, smiled, and calmly defused the situation with, 'Nice try, Willie, you're not fooling me.' She had been exposed to his antics before. What made it all the more funny was that, soon after, a call to see a sick deer was received by reception. The camera crew almost didn't follow to film it as they were convinced it was another hoax.

April 1st may well land at the peak of our rural vetting work, but you'd have to be pretty foolish to think you are ever safe from a prank once that day has been and gone. There have been some memorable gags over the years. Vet Shondie recalls a classic from January a couple of years ago, which also involved a large sea mammal. She was second on-call and heading into the surgery when receptionist Lynda messaged her to say that a sperm whale had arrived in Loch Eriboll and required urgent veterinary assistance. Vet Ken, the first on-call, was already on a calving job, Lynda advised, so Shondie was going to have to take on the leviathan herself. Now, if that sounds well beyond the realm of what someone could credibly fall for, it is worth pointing out that the very same week, a sperm whale had indeed been seen in the loch and was widely reported to have been in some distress and unable to find its way out. The fact that the whale had since left the loch was information Lynda withheld. It was an ideal set-up and Shondie fell for it hook, line and sinker. She texted Lynda in a state of some distress herself: 'What am I going to do with a whale? They're huge! I don't even have a boat!?' before arriving at the surgery to frantically prepare gear for this somewhat oversized patient.

She was, of course, told it was all a big joke before she'd got to the point of driving the 50 miles west to the entirely whale-free loch, but, in a strange twist of fate, Shondie did actually end up attending a large cetacean in real life, who you'll meet later in the summer.

Even the clients couldn't resist a bit of fun at the camera crew's expense. William was scanning pigs for pregnancy one day with cameras in tow. One of the crew was quite obviously very wary of the pigs, distracted from his job and looking around nervously. As the unsettled swine swirled around their feet, one of the farm-hands crept up behind and grabbed the cameraman's leg with a biting pinch of his fingers. He jumped out of his skin and it was nearly the end of a very expensive camera!

I manged to catch out vet William at Christmas once. Every year, without fail, he and I each gratefully received a gift of a bottle of malt whiskey from an elderly couple with greyhounds; it was a way of saying thanks for caring for their animals. Their generosity never went unnoticed by either of us; indeed, it was appreciated with real anticipation – so much so that one year I thought it would be amusing to hide William's bottle, before he'd seen it, but leave my own out on the side in full view. William clearly clocked it instantly, but initially feigned a stoic indifference to the fact he had been forgotten that year by these clients. His body language said it all, though, and after a few days of moping every time he passed my bottle, I eventually showed him where I'd hidden his.

Don't feel sorry for William, though. He is definitely among the chief suspects whenever a prank has been played. His jokes are either infantile or of the type you would certainly not tell in front of infants! And like a big kid, he hides in wait behind doors and obstacles, intent on giving someone the fright of their life when he jumps out on them. The nurses, inevitably, try their best to get their own back. I do wonder what the clients in the consulting rooms must think when they overhear the loud 'boo', followed by screaming.

I've been caught out many times myself. A good one came courtesy of one of our nursing assistants, Michelle. She knew how annoyed I'd get if our expensive, high-quality industrial washing machine broke down. We have a constant stream of soiled bedding from the kennels, and if the machine goes on the blink it is an absolute nightmare as we can't let the stinky stuff pile up, so it all needs to go out to the laundrette. One day she told me the washing machine had a leak. I reacted exactly as expected and walked right into her trap. 'Oh for goodness' sake!' I vented. 'That's ridiculous! We were told they would never go wrong!' I stormed through to the laundry room, fully expecting to see it flooded with water, but instead discovered a leek (the vegetable) sitting in the drum, and all the staff in the know rolling around outside laughing.

As well as a great way of relieving stress, good-natured banter and hijinks really help bind us together as a team, which is vital when the busiest season really starts to sink its teeth in. However, a much more natural lift does arrive in mid-spring too. Easter, for me, heralds the arrival of warmer weather with even more hours of blessed daylight. It is the signal that the wintry half of the spring is gone and the summery half is about to start. *Disclaimer: Not always the case – standard British unpredictable weather applies.* You can even start to imagine a time where the lambing and calving period might finally begin to draw to a close. For now, though, it's still best to get your head down and keep going.

Scientists believe that all modern-day cattle are descendants of the first wild cattle to be domesticated, some 10,000 years ago, in a boomerang-shaped portion of the Middle East known as the Fertile Crescent. They say this half-moon portion of land once stretched from the Nile River on Egypt's Sinai Peninsula all the way to the southern edge of Turkey; it would later become known as the 'Cradle of Civilization'. Fed by luscious wetlands and the fresh waters of the Nile, Euphrates and Tigris rivers, the Fertile Crescent was the perfect place to develop some of the earliest methods of formal farming. According to bones excavated and examined from Iranian archaeological sites, it was the wild – and sadly now extinct – aurochs ox that was most likely the earliest descendent of all the cow breeds we see farmed today.

It is believed that those aurochs in Iran that were successfully domesticated for the very first time probably comprised an initial herd of as few as 80 individuals. Compare that to today, when it is estimated that the global cattle population clears a staggering one billion and consists of over 1,000 recognised breeds.

In Caithness and north Sutherland, the Continental cattle breeds are very popular, particularly the Charolais, the Limousin, the Simmental and, to a lesser extent, the Salers. All of these are often cross-bred with dairy breeds or native beef breeds such as the Beef Shorthorn or our own Aberdeen Angus, which is also kept as a pedigree animal too.

You could be forgiven for wondering, if you were a beef farmer, why you wouldn't always aim to see a huge calf pop out of each cow, to maximise your profits on every animal. Simply put, there is a finite size of hole that the calf must pass through to enter the world. There is a trade-off then, as the larger the calf, the greater the risk of its getting stuck or possibly dying in the process of delivery. Even if a Caesar is successfully performed, the vet's fee cuts into the profit margin for that calf, effectively reducing its value. Better to aim for a calf that stands a good chance of being delivered naturally but which has a rapid growth rate once up and running. Bulls can be selected for siring based on their size and other statistics, if available, such as 'calving ease', which is not an exact science but functions as a guide. Cross-breeding also allows farmers to select the more desirable traits from a mix of breeds, such as the extra muscling that comes with the Belgian Blue breed.

When outsiders think of the cows of the Highlands, it is fair to say that one particular breed of cattle immediately springs to mind. It is, of course, the Highland cow, a proud Scottish icon printed on postcards, keyrings and tea towels in gift shops right across the land. They come in a variety of coat colours, from black to the more familiar red. With their thick, shaggy hair; long, solid horns; and that tufty ginger toupee that flops down from the crown of their head over their big brown eyes, they may well have secured an eternal mainstream appeal among visitors, but the Highland is no softie. It is a very hardy breed, built and bred to withstand the foulest of conditions the Highlands can throw at it. They are extremely self-sufficient creatures too, exceptionally well adapted to living on truly wild, exposed hillsides, and are quite comfortable overwintering outside, while their thicker-set but thinner-coated Continental cousins snuggle up to each other inside barns and byres.

Aside from being a huge tourist draw and a national icon, the Highland does have some commercial appeal for its beef. They are comparatively lean when held up against the more popular commercial beef breeds, but their well-marbled meat can fetch a premium price on the market. The stockier Continental breeds may be more favoured by beef producers, but a Highland-Continental cross might bring the best of both – the former contributing hardiness and an ability to convert rough grazing into muscle and the latter providing size and bulk.

There aren't many pure Highland cow folds up here anymore. A few may be kept alongside a more commercial herd. Those who keep them are mostly doing it for the love of the breed and the role they'll play in preserving its legacy. As such, they are commonly found on crofts and smallholdings run by people who rear them for the joy of it and who have a full-time job doing something else entirely.

The fact there are so few Highland cows up here, combined with all that natural in-built resilience and self-sufficiency, means a vet visit to a Highland cow is a very rare event. This spring, though, Ken did attend such a call-out.

It was a set-up fairly typical of Highland cattle farmers. Martin is a part-time crofter and full-time policeman. He farms in the mornings and evenings after work, and takes his holidays to coincide with the most important duties in his farming calendar. Martin has a small croft that has been passed down through his family since the end of the Second World War, and within his drystone walls he manages a small flock of sheep and his Highland cattle, making him the third generation of his family to take on this iconic breed.

One of Martin's Highland cows had just given birth after a nine-month pregnancy, which, no matter what species you are, is something that puts a heavy toll on the body. In the womb the calf exerts a huge demand on the mother's resources. Plus, there's the physical stress of giving birth itself, and just when you think it's all over, the udder then asks greedily of her system to provide ongoing nourishment for the needy infant. It is not surprising, then, that around the time of calving is a risky juncture for the occurrence of what we call a 'metabolic disorder'. This is when a final growth spurt in the foetus, and the preparation of the udder for milk production, can be overwhelming to the mother. Trouble can strike the cow within a day or two before she passes her calf or soon afterwards; the latter was the case with Martin's cow.

This Highland cow was lying down on a bed of straw in a stone byre when Ken and vet student Lucy arrived. It was clear she was listless, unable to stand and completely lacking in energy to do anything much at all. Even moving her head seemed to be a struggle, let alone getting up to feed her calf, which was lying in the straw near her side. To any vet, this was a 'down-cow' scenario, meaning just that: a cow not so much down in the mouth but, rather, down and not able to get up on her feet. From the fact she had just calved, Ken deduced that she was most likely suffering from a major mineral deficiency and nothing more sinister. Nonetheless, as crofter Martin slid a thick orange rope around his cow's neck, working it up and over her hugely impressive set of horns, Ken opted to examine her to check that she had indeed given birth without any injury or complication.

Ken fired questions at Lucy as he prepared to work. She was in her final year as a student and on the verge of graduation. Lucy was really keen to take a job in a rural mixed practice like ours, and came from a farming background, so was already well grounded in the typical issues suffered by cattle. Still, this Highland cow offered a great example of the kinds of conditions that the calving season can throw up.

It's so important to take students out into the field to witness first-hand the jobs we undertake. Indeed, within reason, and with my support, I try to allow my students to 'get their hands dirty' and even give them a chance to take the lead on the simpler procedures. At university you study a lot of academic theory and see some pretty unusual cases given the specialised hospital setting, but cases are spread thin over a large year-group of students, and the opportunities to see the more common routine ailments can be fairly limited. In the second part of their degree course, veterinary students will spend much of their vacation time gaining experience within vet clinics. It gives them a great chance to put theory into practice and gives us the opportunity to get involved in their development. It is something we all really enjoy.

In her collapsed state, Martin's Highland cow was always going to be easier for Ken to examine than she would have been if she had been stood up over her calf, displaying her full maternal guard and might. Cows have a reputation for being quite docile and plodding in their general daily demeanour, but make no mistake, any cow with young is likely to be very protective. Around calving time, they can display a frightening change in attitude, with real aggression towards anyone, or anything, that they think might be posing a threat to their calf. Indeed, it is one of the many reasons why walkers are discouraged from entering fields containing cows with young calves, especially if they have dogs.

There have been instances in the past where dogs and their owners have been charged, trampled and killed for simply straying into the dangerous space between a cow and her calf. Really, extreme caution should be displayed by any member of the public at any time, but particularly during calving time. Footpaths through fields with cows and calves are best avoided altogether, but if you do find yourself in such a field, the general advice is to stay well away from the herd and walk around them calmly and quietly. Stay close to a boundary that you can leap or scale in desperation, avoiding areas of exposed open field. Keep your dog on a short lead, and if the cows are behaving aggressively, charging or about to charge, head quickly to safety. Be prepared to let go of your dog if you are in imminent danger; a dog is slick and fast and has a far better chance without you, and you certainly have a better chance without the dog.

Nonetheless, as vets, we sometimes have no option but to assume a degree of risk while attending to cows, and, to varying degrees, all of us have picked up bumps, bruises and scars. There are two areas that fundamentally need your attention: the kick zone and the head-butt zone. But you should always be aware that cows are immensely strong beasts with a huge amount of mass. Even if you avoid the head and hooves and place yourself by their sides, you can easily wind up getting crushed against a wall or gate if you're not careful.

Calving is certainly one time when we are naturally in very close proximity to potentially distressed cows. Shondie recalls being hoofed so hard in the thigh by a cow that she actually flew across the pen and landed face down in the straw. Luckily, she was stood close to the cow, so it wasn't able to quite exert maximum bone-shattering force, but she was badly bruised. Vet William also once had his arm broken by a cow when it kicked it hard against a metal fence. And then there's the castration of bull calves.

Some calves are of a pretty substantial size and strength by the time they meet the castrator's blade, so great care must be taken. We often use a piece of machinery called a 'cattle crush' or 'cattle crate' for examining and treating cows. It is essentially a very strong but narrow restraining cage that gives a cow enough room to stand, but not enough room to leap around and cause injury to themselves or us. Vets and farmers have access from outside the crate to examine and treat the animal. Often, the younger cattle don't quite fill it out, leaving side-to-side leeway within the crate. The way we get around that is by getting someone to press up against the calf's body from the inside, effectively pinning it to the side of the crate and restricting its movement. This person holds the tail straight up in the air, as for some reason, that tends to stop the calves kicking quite so much. The in-crate human volunteer, usually a farmhand, is actually in a fairly safe position. However, for the vet standing behind with a scalpel, there's no getting away from the fact that, whatever you do to maintain the calm and immobility of the animal, you are still about to cut off its testicles while positioned right in the firing line of those powerful hind legs.

We very much dissuade farmers from leaving castration until the calves become stirk-sized. A stirk is a large weaned calf, not fully grown but no longer small and easily handled; I sometimes think it's easiest to think of stirks as teenage cattle for this reason! Smaller, placid stirks may be manageable, but having a human in the crate alongside the more sizable and often fractious beasts is best avoided. Such animals are occasionally presented for castration, but generally the younger the calf is presented, the better – for them and for us!

Unfortunately for Ken, a couple of years ago, the farmer on hand had a bad cruciate ligament injury from playing football; so, Ken felt he couldn't really ask him to step into the crush and push up against the stirk. Instead, he just got him to hold it as best he could, and placed a bar behind the beast's rear end to limit his backwards movements. Unfortunately, in hindsight, that bar was a very bad idea. Ken stooped down to make his cut and the stirk hoofed him so hard he broke his arm right up against the bar. That injury was the reason Ken didn't feature too prominently in the first season of *The Highland Vet*, and why his arm was in a sling whenever he did appear. I have already referred to Ken's propensity for on-the-job injury, and as well as the aforementioned horse incident, he has offered his head to the rapidly moving limbs of a cow too.

Probably my own most dramatic career injury was caused by a large calf – a borderline stirk. I've still got the scar to prove it. It took place in the corner of a field just on the edge of town, and I, too, was castrating a batch of substantially sized calves. Despite the fact that the farmers and I were all performing our duties as we should, the calf kicked out with a hind leg at a critical moment and sank the scalpel blade I was holding deep into the back of my hand.

It must have hit an artery, as the blood squirted out of me in an arc some two feet into the air (although that distance increases each time I tell the story). I looked up to the farmers from behind my bovine assailant. 'Well,' I began, while trying to limit blood loss with pressure from my other hand, 'I think that's probably me for today, fellas.' I climbed one of the gates forming the makeshift pen and dashed to my car, handily parked close by in the field.

The benefit of being a vet with a car boot stocked for every eventuality is that I had come prepared to treat any wound or injury, though I had not really imagined having to use my kit on myself! I pulled out a large crepe bandage I kept for horses and wrapped it firmly around my hand, and this thankfully stemmed the blood flow. The farmers didn't seem to know how to help; after all, I was the most qualified person there but, oddly, I was also the patient! 'I'll be alright,' I offered. 'I'll radio in and get someone to come and finish up.' In my early days in Thurso, before mobile phones became mainstream, we used two-way radios to contact the base, and as I had left four and a half calves uncastrated, another vet would need to attend. I jumped into the car and put her in gear, only to discover I was stuck fast in the mud. The farmers did then prove useful in my time of need and pushed my vehicle out of a soggy rut, permitting me to drive myself gingerly to the local hospital, changing gears with a hand compressed in a bloodstained dressing.

The staff at the hospital initially seemed more impressed with the type of bandage we had at our disposal in veterinary medicine rather than the fact my hand had just been sliced open while removing the privates of a calf, but they soon got down to stitching me back up.

I'll never forget the moment I returned to our surgery with my painful and freshly stitched hand neatly wrapped in a somewhat encumbering dressing. Sympathy? *Sympathy?* Not a jot came my way. In those days there was an ethos of *Get a grip and get on with it.* I was too proud to ask, but would anyone offer to cover my forthcoming on-call duty? That night I was back out on the farms and somehow managed to conduct two cow Caesars with one hand partially incapacitated. In addition, 'getting a grip' caused blood to leak into my dressing as I worked. I double-gloved over the bandage and just hoped for the best. I'm sure the doctor who stitched me would have been livid at my blatant disregard for the rule of sensible restricted activity to allow healing. Ah, the good old days! They were certainly different times back then; we'd probably have to give someone a couple of weeks of sick leave or desk duty for that kind of thing today.

The fact that significant injuries by cattle stick in our minds underlies the reality that such events are, on one hand, quite alarming but, on the other hand, thankfully rare. The risk of getting hurt by a cow, stirk or calf on the job is actually very low, especially if you take sensible precautions and work by them. Putting your head near a hoof is not a good idea generally, nor is standing within striking range of the horns of a Highland cow. Collectively, we have worked with thousands of cows during our careers, but the instances of substantial injury remain happily (and going forward, hopefully) few and far between.

The Highland cow being looked after by Ken and Lucy may not have been particularly large when compared to some of the giant Continental breeds, but what they lack in physical stature they more than compensate for with all that intimidating headgear. The thick, sharp curved horns of a Highland cow have points that can often sit a metre apart. Make no mistake: they know exactly where those horns end and exactly how to use them. Highland cows might look superficially sedate, biddable, even cute, but it's safer to treat them with the respect they deserve. Don't for one second think that they couldn't gore you with their armoury in the blink of an eye if, like any breed, they felt threatened or the maternal instinct to protect a calf were evoked. Even if an individual persuades you that she's as calm and cuddly as a toy in a tartan tourist shop, watch those horns! She could simply turn and innocently skewer you with no hostile intentions at all.

The most sensible move is to stay well out of the range of those long horns and to always bear in mind that, even when you think you're safe, it's best not to let your guard down. If you have to do anything clinical around a Highland's face or neck, keep the horns in your peripheral vision, and then make sure the cow's head is appropriately restrained before doing anything else. Having successfully secured a rope around this Highland's neck, Ken loaned further control of her sharp end by fitting a halter over her nose and head. Crofter Martin then tethered the halter's free lead rope to a very solid steel rail on the perimeter of the enclosure.

Lucy listened to the patient's heart with her stethoscope and found there were no cardiovascular concerns, before Ken inserted his gloved arm into the cow's vagina to assess all was well after passing her calf. He pulled out the afterbirth, a huge, dark fluid-filled sac, which spilled its contents into the straw bedding as his fingers tore the membranes. Nothing unusual there. With the rest of Ken's examination confirming there had been no injury sustained during birth, and no obvious signs of infection, his presumptive diagnosis was a mineral deficiency and so he began immediate treatment.

A common and classic cause of a 'down cow' around the time of calving is a deficiency of the essential mineral calcium. Before research shed light on the underlying cause, this syndrome was labelled 'milk fever', a name we still use today, because of the obvious association with the burgeoning udder. Indeed, this clear link led to quite a bizarre-sounding treatment to be used in days of old, before it had been worked out that low bodily calcium was the culprit. The udder was pumped up by a pneumatic pump; I've heard that people even improvised with a bicycle pump! I can only imagine that the old-time vets' and farmers' logic was aimed at reducing milk production. More surprising than the technique itself is that it did appear to significantly improve the condition! Interestingly, later research found evidence of increased calcium levels in the blood after pumping. The pump pressure is postulated to have somehow forced calcium from the milk back into the bloodstream. However, although there were claims of doing little harm, farmers, please don't run for the bicycle pump next time you see this condition. Modern treatment is slick, quick and safe.

Calcium is required in the body for a multitude of different functions, but the one critical to the debilitating condition being experienced by Martin's Highland was its role in muscle contraction. Without enough calcium, the cow's skeletal muscles lacked the strength to allow her to rise to her hooves. In more advanced cases, the heart muscle becomes unable to circulate blood properly, and you'll also see swelling of the abdomen as the stomach fills with gas due to failing gut muscles.

Calcium levels do fluctuate naturally within the body of a cow, but the massive calcium demand to provide for growth of the calf's bones in the final stages of pregnancy, plus that ploughed into the udder for making milk, had clearly depleted the reserves of this recumbent Highland mum. A cow's food intake may drop temporarily as calving approaches, so, before you know it, the calcium level in a cow's body can quickly slide from being just enough to so little that she finds herself on the brink of death unless something is done. When the cow gets to the point that she is unable to rise, her calcium level is already so critically low that it will not rebound again naturally. Left untreated, the heart becomes so weak, and the ballooning guts place so much pressure on the vascular system, that she will eventually just die of circulatory failure. If this occurs prior to calving, the consequences for any onboard dependents are all too obvious.

One or two 400ml bottles of calcium solution is a good starting point when presented with this condition. Ken's experience had allowed him to pre-empt this diagnosis and he already had bottles warming in a bucket of hot water. Next, he slid two large-bore needles under the skin over the cow's ribcage on either side of her chest. Ideally, you'd look to run the calcium into one of the cow's jugular veins, but these are in the neck and, thanks to those horns, Ken decided this was perhaps best left as a no-go zone.

A flutter valve was used, which allows fluid to drain by gravity, at speed, from a bottle down a length of tubing into the cow. With a helping hand from vet student Lucy, Ken was then able to run two bottles of concentrated mineral solution simultaneously into their patient. It took five minutes of Ken and Lucy acting as human drip stands to completely drain the bottles under the cow's skin. Raising the bottle above head height increases the effect of gravity on the flow rate. Personally, as I do this, I swap the bottle from arm to arm as muscle ache sets in. Then they gave the whole area a really good massage, to get the calcium solution to disperse and absorb into the deficient body as rapidly as possible.

With the vital calcium now working its way into her system, the next step was to take care of this Highland's newborn calf. She was only a little over an hour old, and had already made it to her feet for a few wobbly first steps around the straw; but, on account of the state of her mum, getting her all-important first drink of milk had been somewhat delayed.

The first milk a mum produces is a unique fluid called 'colostrum'. It's a dense and thick cream-like substance rich with nutrients and antibodies. These antibodies cross from the calf's bowel into its bloodstream and remain effective for around three months, providing crucial 'borrowed' immunity to disease as the young animal builds its own immune system. The bowel is only capable of making this transfer for a short while after birth, thus there is a narrow window of opportunity to ensure that a newborn calf receives its important first meal. This is considered to be four to six hours; from there, antibody absorption declines quickly. Delayed or inadequate colostrum intake will very much increase the chance of a calf dying from disease within the first few weeks of life.

With the cow still unable to support her half-ton body weight, Ken and Lucy began to milk her teats into a large plastic jug as she lay in the straw. The colostrum flowed easily and was then transferred into a bottle to be hand-fed to the calf. With that problem successfully resolved, it quickly became apparent that the health status of the mother was already shifting significantly for the better.

About ten minutes after the administration of the medication, the cow began to really burp. Her stomach muscles were engaging again and she was beginning to get rid of the gas that had built up within her. Her abdomen began to shrink as the belching continued, and, as Ken and Lucy edged away, she was already beginning to look a whole lot more alert. Ken left to prepare some additional oral fluids to give to her; however, in just the time it took for him to walk to the boot of his car and back, she was ready to make an attempt to stand. More slowly than normal and with a slight stagger, the revitalised patient arose and was most definitely not appreciating the fact she was being restrained by a short length of rope. Crofter Martin only just managed to remove one rope from around her neck before she went powering off across her enclosure, warding off all interlopers from her furry little daughter and firmly exerting her maternal authority.

It was a very good sign indeed, and Ken wisely decided it was best to abandon his own rope halter, still wrapped around the hairy head sporting those – now upwardly mobile – lethal weapons. A violent rebuke from the cow was likely, and could prove very dangerous; they all agreed the halter could be retrieved when she calmed down.

If you have never witnessed it first-hand, the turnaround from treatment for calcium deficiency in a cow can appear really quite miraculous. This Highland had gone from being lethargic and immobile when Ken and Lucy had arrived, to bristling with attitude and back to full-strength within just half an hour.

From a rural vet's perspective, this has to be one of the most impressive fixes we ever get to pull off.

Chapter Eleven

All Hail Caesar!

May has arrived in Caithness and an early-summer sunshine has swept in with it.

For many wildlife species, the breeding season has already begun in earnest. The puffin colonies have reassembled on Dunnet Head's clifftops, excavating nesting burrows in the soil, or settling into crags and cavities in the rock, before laying their single precious egg. The wide-open marshes and peatlands of the Flow Country may see greenshank, dunlin, and golden plover with their chicks, alongside many other young waders and wild-fowl. All of them keen to feed and fatten on the wide profusion of invertebrate life breaking free from chrysalis, case or egg.

In the rivers, lochs and estuary edges, the secretive otters breed and give birth to their young, as do the Scottish wildcats in our woodlands. These enigmatic felines are so elusive, they are almost mythological; we have had only a handful of probable sightings in the very quietest corners of our forests.

For the very keenest of our wildlife observers, the calming seas give way to the spotting of dolphins, porpoises and the very occasional pod of orcas; and there is a palpable lift in the moods of humans across Caithness and north Sutherland too.

You can't really overstate what a consistent period of warm weather and daylight does for the soul. In May we might still have a few lambings coming to the surgery, or a farmer bringing in the odd sick calf. What is really lovely is that, when they do, we actually get to work in the sunshine and fresh air, right out of the back of the farmer's trailer, instead of having to haul animals into our lambing shed.

It is a foretaste of what is still to come in summer: outdoor work without getting freezing cold, wet or covered in mud (well, not *all* of the time at least!), with everyone feeling so much cheerier and jollier. The surgery can serve as a social hub for farmers too. We'll see them having a good laugh and a catch-up in our car park, nattering to one another long after the purpose of their visit has been fulfilled.

Every vet at the practice will have done their fair share of calving and lambing work by the time May comes around. Don't forget, either, that it isn't as if we can hit the pause button on all the pet animal work in the surgery. That all has to carry on as normal, and it is incredible how often a really tough night of calving coincides with a challenging nocturnal feline or canine catastrophe.

Although each vet, each year, will work their way randomly through the list of birthing malpresentations I have previously outlined, once the peak of lambing is over, a fair part of the farm emergency work revolves around calves that are simply too big for their mums. Sometimes the extra pull of our calving jack will solve the problem, but Caesars are a frequent daily, and nightly, occurrence. The big discernment and responsibility sits squarely with the vet: will it be a squeezer or a Caesar?

Common offenders are heifers (young cows in their first pregnancy, who are still growing as their foetuses grow inside them too). Another factor is that some breeds have a longer gestation period; for example, the Charolais and Simmental can have calves in the womb for heading towards ten months, whereas other breeds fall between nine and nine and a half. This extra two or three weeks of growth can make a huge difference to the size and stockiness of a calf. Nourishment during pregnancy also plays a role in producing an oversized foetus, although it is a little more complex than simply 'more food, big calf', even if that often seems to be the case. Nature tends to prioritise propagation of the species and so protects pregnancy. A poorly nourished cow will 'burn it off her own back' to produce a healthy calf; I have seen many a thin cow deliver a whopper. But it can certainly be said that managing a cow's nutrition throughout pregnancy is very important.

No matter the underlying cause, though, the consequence of a cow's dystocia will often involve the vet reaching for his scalpel.

Amid the chaotic call-outs and death-defying saves of the calving season, there are always a few moments where memories are created. Some can really be quite heart-warming.

One morning when my daughters were very young, I was called 'out west' to Ted's croft, which was about an hour from the Thurso practice. A cow was calving and needed assistance. It wasn't an unusual call and, as it turned out, not an unusual calving; I delivered the new little heifer calf with the aid of my trusty calving jack and then Ted and I stood back to admire the wonders of nature as the mum licked her new babe.

All cattle, by law, are ear-tagged with an individual number, and some farmers have an impressive recognition of each cow and can tell you their numbers before a tag is close enough to be legible, even in quite a large herd. But how much more friendly to give them names. It seems the smaller the farm, the more likely a cow is to have a name. This was one such place and, as the man of the moment, I was given the privilege of naming the newborn.

I pondered for a few seconds and then offered the name Brianna, after our first daughter. That evening I would then have the pleasure of telling her that she had a cute little calf on a croft as a namesake. After the events of that day, of course, I'd bump into Ted from time to time and I would make sure I asked how Brianna was getting on.

About three years later, I answered the phone one breakfast time to hear Ted's out-of-place Lancastrian accent asking once again for assistance with a heifer struggling to calve. Technically I should have sent the first on-call vet, as I was the second, but the first vet would not have thanked me for sending them on a two-to-three-hour round trip when they were due to clock off in half an hour! As second on-call vet, I was scheduled to continue with a day's work, and besides, a trip towards the mountains and scattered crofts of Sutherland – not to mention Ted's croft, nestled in a pleasant wee green valley running into a sea cove – is always a bit of a draw for me.

As I pulled on my waterproofs by his small byre, I asked Ted what the problem was. 'It's Brianna,' he said, 'she's a bit tight with her first calf.'

There she was, my little Brianna, all fully grown and now about to become a mother herself. As a heifer, this was her first experience of giving birth, and I was more than happy to offer my help. (But please note, I hope that the appropriate midwives and obstetricians will be on hand when Brianna, the human, provides me with a grandchild!)

Just like her mother, only a little assistance was required before a pretty wee calf was lying beside her, ready to be lovingly licked clean. Admiring the scene once more, Ted and I discussed the naming of the new arrival. Of course, there was really only one option for me: I chose Cara, the name of our other daughter.

I took a photo on the basic mobile phone I possessed in those days. It wasn't great quality by modern smartphone standards, but it was good enough to print and write a short paragraph of explanation underneath for my girls to take to school as a more unusual item for the weekly show-and-tell.

Vets vie each year for their claim on the worst night duty with respect to workload, and believe me, there have been some stinkers! When it came to awarding a prize for the single toughest night-time calf delivery this year, Ken was certainly up there with a job he admits was one of the most taxing of his career to date.

It all began as a typical evening call. Ken climbed into his bed in the classic state of mental purgatory experienced by all on-call rural vets during spring: do I stay up in the knowledge that the phone will probably ring soon and that it's best to be alert and ready? Or do I try and get some sleep, just in case it doesn't ring for a few hours and this is my only shot at getting some rest? Our old friend Murphy has a law about such things whereby if you opt for the former you end up sitting awake for hours when you could've been asleep, and if you go for the latter, you get woken just after you've dropped off, which is the absolute pits.

Ken opted for a halfway house by taking a book to bed, but at 9.45pm his home phone rang anyway. For those of us, like Ken, who have a fair few calving seasons under our belt, rational thought can be supplanted by a strange sense of foreboding at times like this. Before his partner, Catherine, had even answered, a chill had invaded Ken's warm and cosy bed. This was going to be a big one, he could just feel it.

'Ken,' Catherine called across the hall. Even the tone of her voice had said most of what he needed to know. Only the location was required. 'It's a calving out at Brackside Farm.' Ken knew the place well. Brackside was farmed by Will Sutherland and his son Liam. Both were very experienced farmers who maintained a herd that was generally well able to calve naturally. Will and Liam were also plenty capable of fixing a routine malpresentation themselves; a call-out to Brackside was rare. So rare in fact, that despite his 16 years at the practice, this was Ken's first ever calving job there.

Ken soon had the details: it was a four-year-old Simmental cow with a suspected twisted womb, and as he hauled himself out of bed, he highly suspected he wouldn't be seeing home again for a number of hours.

Brackside sits around 12 miles west of Thurso, out by the village of Reay. As Ken got ready, he called the *Highland Vet* camera crew to advise them that this would likely be a story they'd want to follow (having first checked with farmer Will that he didn't mind the job being filmed) and then jumped into his car.

Thoughts and feelings can evolve quickly on the drive out to a potentially difficult job. For Ken that night, he went from feeling a bit sick, cold and grumpy to beginning to visualise and prepare for what he had coming up. As he drove, he made a mental checklist of the gear he'd need, the medicines and surgical kit, before pondering what the presentation might look like along with the various steps he would need to take to correct it.

By the time Ken arrived at Brackside, he was ready to roll, as were the camera crew.

Farmer Will was stood beneath a pool of gold thrown out by the electrical lighting in his calving shed. Behind a pair of thick-rimmed spectacles, he was, quite clearly, very concerned about the predicament of his cow.

'An awkward one here,' he began, leaning over the steel railing and looking in on the thick head of his Simmental. 'I don't know how long she's been at it.' He turned away and paced across the shed as the TV camera captured him narrating his thoughts. 'The calf's lying the wrong way.' He gestured with the upturned palm of his hand to show the position.

On the concrete flooring outside the cattle shed, Ken kicked off his shoes and took off his jacket, before pulling on his waterproof trousers and a short-sleeved top over thin disposable arm-length gloves. It may have been spring, but there was still a bite in the air on this Highland night. Short sleeves may be practical when working in a cow's rear, but Ken opted to pull a bobble hat over the crown of his head for at least a little extra warmth.

The cow herself was restrained behind a calving gate, with her solid head secured at one end in a locking yoke. Will and Liam pressed the gate against her side; too much sideways wiggle room would not make Ken's examination easy and might risk damaging his arm.

Ken gleaned some more information from her owner. Will felt the cow had been quite uncomfortable and increasingly in pain for some time. He added that there hadn't been any signs that her labour was progressing at all.

Often, by this stage of a calving, you'd expect to see a bit of the placenta starting to appear at the cow's vulva. Her waters should then break, and then the feet and perhaps a nose of the calf start to present. The cow behind the gate was showing absolutely none of that, but she was kicking at her belly, a sure sign of abdominal discomfort.

Such a lack of visible progress is usually a very good external indicator that there is likely to be either a significant malpresentation or a restriction such as a twisted womb. Will had had a feel prior to Ken's arrival and sensed there was possibly a uterine twist from just how tight it was in there, but he'd really struggled to lay his fingers properly on the calf.

Ken slid his hand inside the cow. She mooed angrily and the gate started to shake and clank as she tried to shuffle side to side. Will's earlier deduction was right. 'The calf is completely on its back,' began Ken, as he tried to feel around for more information. 'It's just difficult to tell ... Yeah, twisted womb as well. It's not very open.' The cow rattled the gate with force. 'Easy, girl,' said Ken calmly, as he shifted and struggled to get a different angle on the calf wedged inside.

Will massaged the great ginger back of his prized animal as Ken worked away. 'It's really tricky.' Ken started to huff, 'There's just not enough room to get in there, and it's a big calf as well,

I think. It's completely upside down, with its feet sticking up above it.'

Ken soon confirmed, beyond any doubt, that the reason the calf was presenting upside down was because the womb itself was badly twisted. To remind you briefly of the main aspects of this scenario: if we use the balloon image for the uterus, with the calf lying within, then it has all rotated, creating a twist in the balloon's neck. This twist narrows the exit from the uterus and, in this case, has left the calf flipped right over.

When you initially put your arm inside a cow with a twist, it might feel like not much at all is happening; you just get a sense that something is amiss. But Ken, by rummaging and contorting, managed to assess the calf's presentation and also detected a corkscrew shape in the cow's birth canal.

With the problem diagnosed, the next step is to decide what you can practically do to solve it. As previously mentioned, in a cow, surgery might be avoided if you are able to untwist it by hand. You slide your hand in through the corkscrewed region, grip the calf by whatever you can find – be it a leg, a shoulder or the side of its head – and do a bit of Scottish country dancing behind the cow to impart momentum to the womb. Get it swinging and, with some luck, you might just get the whole uterus to go all the way over and achieve a natural birth.

That is no mean feat. So much is working against you. As methods go, it is probably a fifty-fifty, but it is well worth a go to spare the cow (and the vet in the middle of the night) the ordeal of a Caesar. In the yellow light of the shed, Ken gave it all he had. He rocked his arm backwards and forwards, exerting himself and gaining a little swinging motion. As he fatigued, he swapped from his left arm to his right, but ultimately, it was to no avail.

With his sleeves and gloves coated in bloody fluid, he took a deep breath and admitted to Will and the camera that it had him beat. 'You can move it a little bit, but it just flops right back down again. It's quite heavy.'

After 20 minutes of sustained effort, Ken was quite physically exhausted. In spite of the unfavourable odds, you always feel dispirited when you can't pull it off and untwist the womb. It shouldn't be the case, but it can feel like a personal failure. Yet there's more at stake than your pride. Time is not your friend when it comes to a twisted womb. The twist can badly constrict the blood vessels that supply the uterus; these are like small hosepipes, such is the demand by a growing calf at the end of pregnancy. Obstruction of these vessels will lead to damage of the uterine tissue, starvation of the unborn calf's oxygen, and then death.

Every single minute that passes without a resolution to the twist counts against the calf's chances of survival, and even its mum's. If Will hadn't come out to his shed that night to check on her, then the chances of the calf still being alive in the morning would have been very slim. There are times when a vet will be called to fix a twisted womb but the calf will, unfortunately, have already passed away.

It takes real diligence and experience on the farmers' part to watch their cows day and night during calving time, just so they can spot the smallest of signs that a problem might be arising. Remember, thanks to her twisted womb, there were very few visibly obvious signs that Will's cow was in labour at all. In such situations a farmer can only rely on subtle behavioural signs:

the cow not interacting with the rest of the herd, eating less, kicking and nuzzling around in her straw bedding, taking an overkeen interest in young calves of other mothers, holding her tail in a persistently elevated position and possibly dribbling milk from her teats.

In some cows it might be quite obvious there is a problem, especially if they are lying down and groaning, but in many, it really does just come down to the skills of the stockperson to know when one of their animals is not quite right. Will is one of those farmers, and such attentive livestock keepers tend to do the best at calving time. Even if they have a herd of hundreds, they are able to see the metaphorical wood for the trees, isolate an individual that's struggling and initiate a timely emergency call-out.

With the procedure plainly impossible by manipulation via the birth canal, the only option left to Ken was to go for what farmers often refer to as the 'side door': an emergency Caesar. He asked Will for consent, which he naturally granted immediately: 'It has to be done. It can't stay where it is!'

Ken has undertaken several hundred caesareans throughout his time at Thurso. In calving season, they are routine procedures, and he was emboldened by the fact that this cow was well secured by a yoke and a calving gate, and that the farm building was very clean by many farms' standards.

He popped open a plastic DIY toolbox containing syringes, medicine bottles, and his surgical instruments. The hair was clipped from her left flank and local anaesthetic was injected to knock out sensation to the area to be incised. Then, to limit the risk of infection, he thoroughly scrubbed the area, plus his own arms, with a surgical antiseptic detergent. It may seem strange to us as humans, but the plan is that the cow stays standing and fully conscious throughout.

Ken's incision in the cow's left abdominal wall was, by necessity, about 40cm long running vertically, situated halfway between her ribs and her pelvis. Generally, with cow Caesars about 20 per cent of your time is spent getting to the point when the calf is lying on the straw beside you. Then the rest is spent making sure you've sutured the cow properly. You've got to make sure the womb is completely watertight first, then reconstruct the three abdominal muscle layers you'd cut through, and finally stitch the skin, which, perhaps unsurprisingly, can be almost as tough as leather. I have found that visitors to a farm, perhaps friends or family, often want to watch a Caesar, and they find the whole thing riveting initially, but soon lose interest once they realise that the stitching will drag on for a while.

However, with Will's cow, Ken knew this was likely to be a more complicated caesarean delivery than usual. In the majority of cases, you'll find the calf lying in the uterus on the left-hand side of the abdomen with its back legs not too far from your incision; this is one reason why we tend to operate on the mother's left. With one arm in the cow's abdomen up to your shoulder, you press her huge stomach to one side with your elbow and, using only your tactile sense, find the calf's back feet. The calf, still encased in the muscular uterus, is a heavy thing to support with the grip of one hand, but you must pull it up to the gaping hole in the cow's side, then make an incision into the uterus and haul the calf out, usually after passing its feet to a farmhand to help with the pull.

With a twisted womb, you can be fairly confident that the calf isn't going to be in the anticipated position, but this cow took that concept to an extreme. Ken immediately discovered the calf was positioned as far away from him as possible. Moreover, the natural 'handles' – the calf's limbs – were facing away from him. On top of this, it was apparent that the calf was a thumper and, of course, the twist in the womb just added insult to injury. Could anything else make the situation worse?

'She's got a tummy full of food!' Ken exclaimed in dismay. Cows weren't designed with spare room for manoeuvre inside. Organs are packed against organs, all the more so with an enormously full uterus at the end of pregnancy. Remember, the cow's stomach is a monstrous fermentation vat, perhaps 100kg. It is not always an impeding presence during a Caesar, but occasionally it decides to just sit on or against the uterus, making surgical access an absolute nightmare. Ken, already tired from his earlier attempts at untwisting the womb, gripped his surgical scissors in his teeth as he switched positions and arms in an attempt to make headway. He needed to rotate the calf-filled womb against the weight of the heavy stomach, essentially correcting the twist from the worst possible position with everything stacked against him.

Ken is not a small man. He's tall with broad shoulders and a body kept in shape by an active job and a regular bit of circuit training, but, by his own admission, the manoeuvring pushed him right to the edge of his physical capabilities. The lack of space and access meant no one else could scrub in and help out. This was his problem to solve alone. It's worth understanding, too, that this isn't a job where you can make some incremental gains and then take a breather: you either pull the move off in one go or you don't pull it off at all.

After failing at untwisting the womb via the birth canal, a Caesar was supposed to be the easy option. Why didn't it feel like it?! Now, both arms in deep up to his oxters, he pressed so hard into the open abdominal cavity that his feet slid through the hay beneath him like a front-row rugby forward churning up grass on a wet day at Murrayfield. At last! Ken managed to gain purchase with one hand on the calf's hip and the other on its chest, and began to heave it up and around with its mum's full stomach bearing right down on top of it.

It had got to the point where Ken was beginning to consider the ridiculous notion that he might have to back out of the cow, stitch her back up again, and then open her up on the right-hand side, when finally, mercifully, he managed to flip the calf and successfully untwist the womb.

All told, Ken guesses he was in the side of that cow for at least an hour, which by anyone's reckoning was a serious workout, especially when you consider that an average Caesar, from the first cut to the final stitch, usually takes less than 40 minutes to complete.

Despite the nip in the air, sweat was pouring from Ken's forehead. His bobble hat certainly seemed surplus to requirements, but the calf was at least now positioned in a place where he was able to make the delivery.

They were not out of the woods, though – not yet at least. After such a long period of time, and so much pressure and stress on mum and calf, there was a real chance that this calf may have died. Stillborn calves are always upsetting, but when you've worked so hard, for so long, to save one, it is truly a sickening feeling. Thoughts were spinning through Ken's mind. Had the womb been twisted for too long? Had the calf suffocated due to delayed access to the vital fresh air? Was all his sweat and exertion to save this life going to have been in vain?

He made an incision in the uterus beside the calf's back legs and passed the hefty limbs to Liam to assist with the pull. 'Please be alive after all that,' Ken pleaded with the calf as it landed in the straw. It twitched the second it touched down – a good sign – and Ken immediately began massaging its side with one hand while clearing out its nostrils with the other.

Suddenly, it snorted mucus out of its great white snout, and before Ken had even finished stitching his mum back together, this young bull was wobbling around, up on his hooves.

In normal circumstances, it can be a little annoying to have a newborn calf staggering around and stumbling into you as you're stitching up; it is not uncommon for them to send a bucket, or your tray of surgical instruments, flying. But as Ken finished up the Caesar, everyone was just immensely glad to see this wee young life tottering in the hay.

For farmers like Will, this whole process would have started with hopeful anticipation of yet another uneventful, unassisted natural birth when the cow first went out to the bull a little over nine months ago; for Ken it started with a worrying phone call a little before 10pm that night. But as they all washed themselves down with the shed's hose, sharing the crack and smiling for the first time in a couple of hours, the sense of relief was enormous.

'I can honestly say that was one of the most challenging caesareans I've done in years,' said Ken, in his closing piece to the camera that he'd almost regretted inviting out on that occasion. 'It was really, *really* difficult.'

He pulled his hose-cleaned waterproof top off his torso, tired but immensely happy. He would head home and attempt to get some well-earned sleep, but at calving time, it was unlikely that this would be his only call of the night.

No matter how demanding the last job was, you can't turn down the next on the basis that you're feeling tired. It's the pact we make, and the deal we must accept, as rural vets. 'Bedtime when you're on call in the spring is a kind of loosely defined thing,' continued Ken, seemingly aging by the minute. 'If you get to your bed and stay there for a few hours, you're quids in! But if you get woken up about half an hour after you get in your bed, well, then you're very depressed!' He chuckled, before jumping back in his car.

Days later the crew picked up with farmer Will, happily stood back in his cattle shed with his cow and her fair-haired newborn bull. 'If Ken hadn't been able to untwist that womb and get that calf out, they'd both be dead by now.' With hands in his pockets, Will nodded in the direction of the cow and calf. 'It's not often this happens, and I don't want it to happen again!'

He started to laugh. In spite of the long nights and uncertainties inherent in the beef industry, Will is a man who just loves his work.

'I actually treat it like a big hobby now. I only regret I hadn't started sooner,' he muses. 'I should never have been an electrician, but my wife says different.' He smiled, before adding, 'Because she says she married an electrician, not a farmer!'

Chapter Twelve

To Be Frank

The veterinary practice in Caithness has always enjoyed a good reputation and has been progressive in its approach to providing veterinary services – a legacy from the 'old boys', which I sense is still running in the veins of the younger generation now at the helm. Change can often come quickly, but at other times it filters in slowly and is apparent only when one reflects back to a former epoque.

'Cleaning cows' would fit this latter category. To be clear, I am not referring to putting a showerhead on the end of a hose and grabbing a bottle of bovine shampoo. When I was in other parts of the country as a student, it was also known by the similar term 'cleansing' a cow. Whatever the terminology, we are referring to the removal of the afterbirth – the placenta – which has been retained after calving.

Cows normally pass the afterbirth within minutes, hours, or at worse, a day or two after giving birth, but occasionally the placenta can literally 'hang around' for several days, even beyond a week. For this period, it dangles from the birth canal, frequently tickling the ground and soiling the cow's legs. Apart from being unsightly, it starts to decompose, and it stinks – really stinks!

The placentae of cows and sheep are not diffusely attached across the whole interior surface of the womb; they attach at multiple discrete sites resembling large buttons, called 'cotyledons'. Removing the afterbirth manually involves a full-length arm into the birth canal whereby we 'unbutton' these placental attachments and apply gentle traction until the whole rotting mess tumbles to the ground.

The passing of the afterbirth is known as the third stage of labour in all common mammals. Our second daughter, Cara, was born in the hospital in Wick. The labour was protracted and utterly exhausting. Indeed, I believe my wife found it quite tiring too. Ridiculous as it may sound, considering I dealt with obstetrics as part of my job and I'd already experienced the birth of our other daughter, I hadn't anticipated the sheer frustration and tedium of this third stage.

Just when we thought it was all over and we could both rest and enjoy the new bundle of joy lying beside us, the midwife got all excited about Jennifer relieving herself of the afterbirth. It was just hanging around. *Get on with it!* I thought. Could it not just come away and let us all relax? The midwife was not at all impressed with my suggestion of applying traction. Just as well I hadn't offered to attach ropes to my daughter's legs to speed up her entrance into the world!

In cows, there had been a general rule passed from generation to generation that after three days, if an afterbirth was still tenaciously trailing at the cow's back end, a vet should attend and remove it. Indeed, a common feature of the profession's day work would be calls, on day three, to visit a farm to do 'the necessary'. I expect James Herriot himself worked by this rule.

However, my generation at university were being taught a radical, subversive, newfangled theory that flew in the face of this received wisdom from antiquity. Although not the case in other species, in cows, the latest knowledge informed us that there was no need to forcibly remove the placenta in almost all cases. Smelly and unsightly though it may be, we were told to just leave it to come away itself, even if it took a week or more. Why intervene unnecessarily and risk damaging the womb if the afterbirth was still stuck fast to the buttons? If a very occasional cow became ill, then removal might be necessary; but that may occur well after the three-day mark, in which case the job would be much easier to complete due to the progression of the decomposition.

When I arrived in Caithness, this way of thinking was a few years old, but such notions can take time to filter into mainstream work and particularly into the expectations of the farming community. Livestock keepers expected their cows to be cleaned and, understandably, wanted the smelly dangly bits out of their lives. Even vets can be cautious about change: what if a cow got sick after we'd refused to remove its afterbirth? It would reflect badly on us, which could be bad for business.

Yet nowadays we seldom get calls to clean cows; I can't recall the last time I did it. Experience over the last couple of decades has proven the theory to be sound.

Frank was a larger-than-life character, a widely respected vet and my boss during my early days in Thurso. His workload was 99 per cent farm animals, with some equine patients, though he tended adeptly to the pet clients when called out of hours. One day, while I was operating on a dog, Frank appeared in the operating room. His countenance was stern. I'd seen that expression before and so braced myself.

He vented his wrath at me. 'Who is telling clients we don't clean cows anymore?' I could imagine steam coming from his ears. I had no escape; I was mid-op and was responsible for my patient. With no opportunity for me to defend myself, the tirade continued.

I could understand his stance, though not his outrage. As an owner of the business, among other implied reasons such as 'you should do as you're told', he cited the *what if* scenario: what if the worst happened and we had said no to a farmer who'd asked for his prize cow to be cleaned? After a couple of futile attempts to say my piece, I accepted my place as an underling and opted to just keep my head down, concentrate on the operation and let it pass.

You see, the thing that bugged me is, for all I know, I could have been dropped in it by another young vet. I had never told a farmer that we no longer cleaned cows. Although, what I frequently did was make small talk, arm in cow, as the stinky juices squelched down my waterproofs. (Incidentally, despite doubling up on arm-length gloves, the stench would still percolate through to your skin and remain for the rest of the day. I feel for the vets-of-old before such gloves were readily available!)

I was merely informing farmers that cleaning cows was out of vogue, and it had been shown to be unnecessary in most cases of retained placenta. Client education is a far cry from refusal to do the job.

One morning, a matter of only weeks later, all the work on the diary had been divided up between the available vets, but there wasn't quite enough to go round. Frank found himself with no calls and seemed to be relishing the opportunity for some well-earned

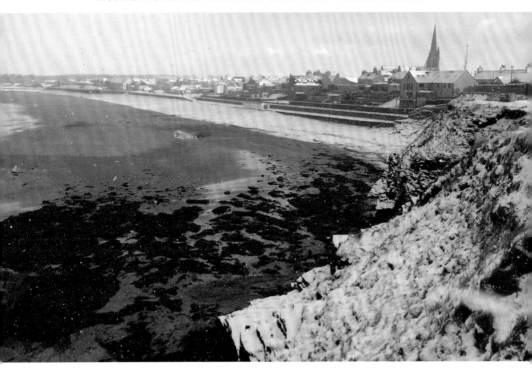

Thurso in the snow

Reay Harbour, Caithness

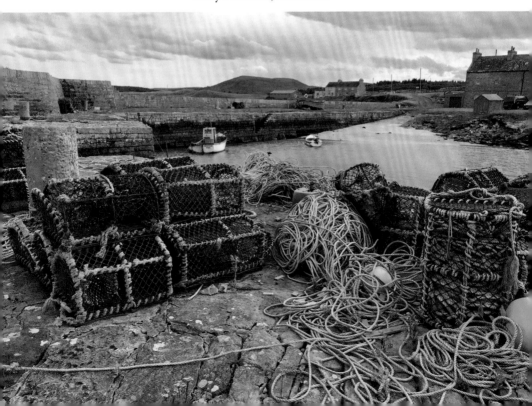

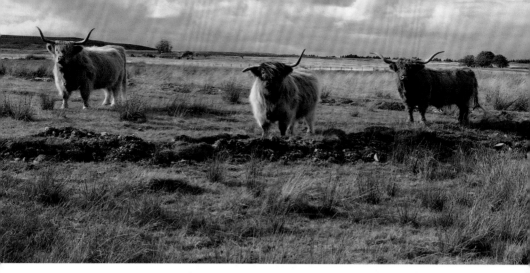

You are never too far from livestock around here,
cows and sheep especially fill the landscape

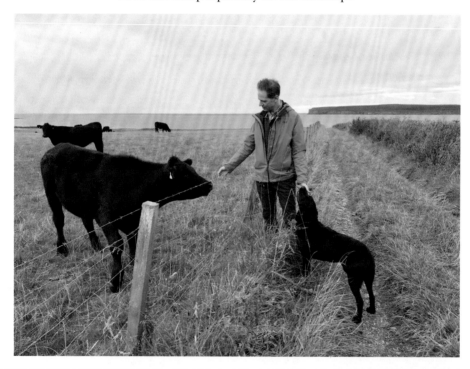

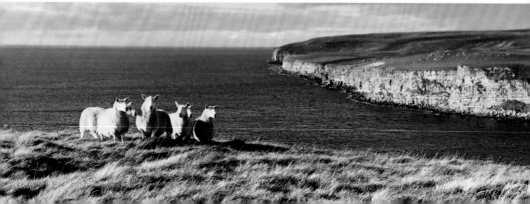

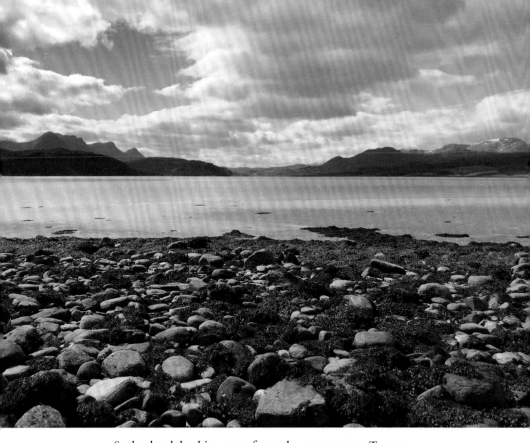

Sutherland, looking west from the causeway at Tongue

Strathy Beach

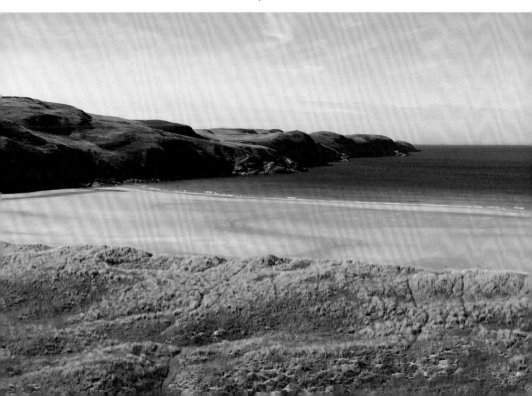

FAMILY - THEN AND NOW!

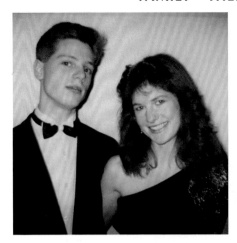

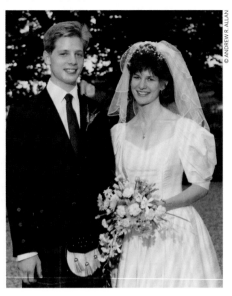

The first vet school ball Jennifer
and I attended together

Our wedding day, September 1992

With our daughters, Brianna and Cara, in Caithness, 2019,
shortly before Brianna's wedding

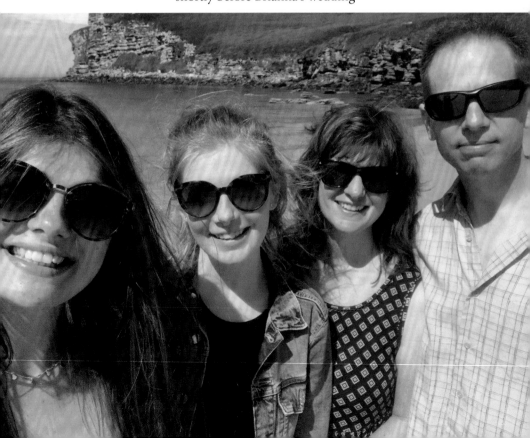

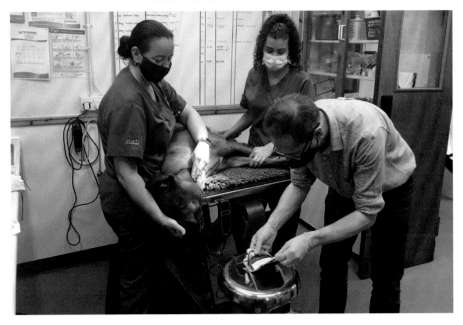

With nurses Caz and Caitlin at the surgery.
Here Caz's dog Obi is kindly acting as a blood donor

The aftermath of fixing a uterine prolapse. The cow went on to do well

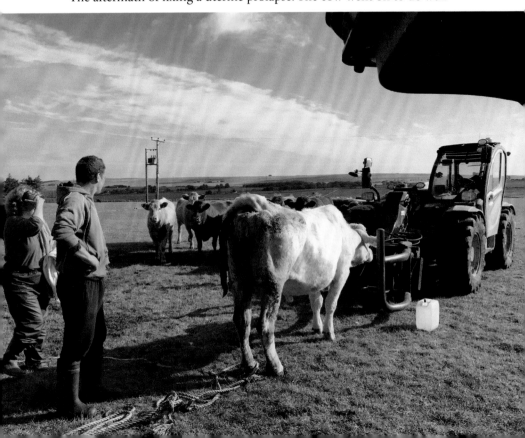

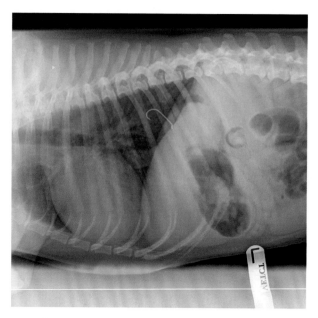

The X-ray that showed us the alarming barbed
fish hook stuck fast in a dog's oesophagus

Here I am treating an abscess in a bull's toe with a
powered grinder (protective gear very necessary!)

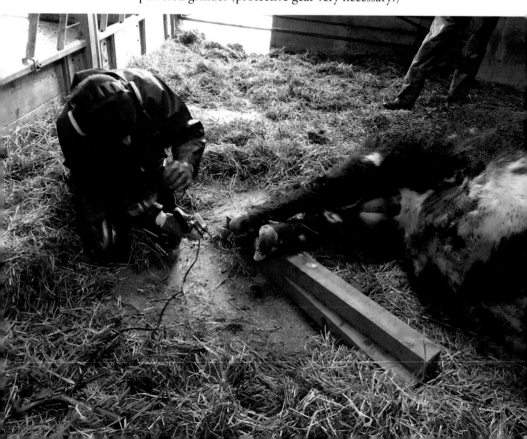

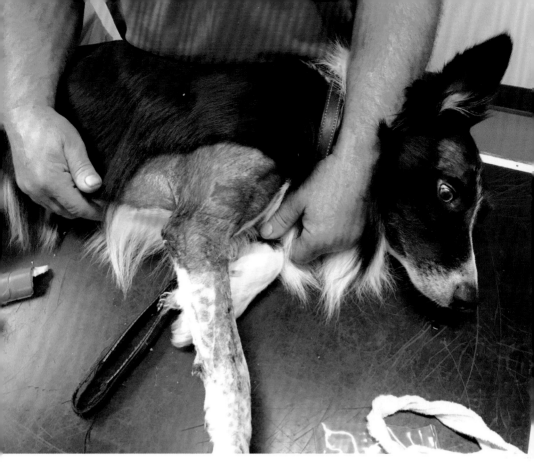

Sweep, the sheepdog who made a remarkable
recovery after running in front of a bus

Bodysuits are handy for cats and dogs to cover wounds after surgery.
We improvised this one for a hamster, but she wasn't as impressed
as we were with ourselves; she slipped it off later that day!

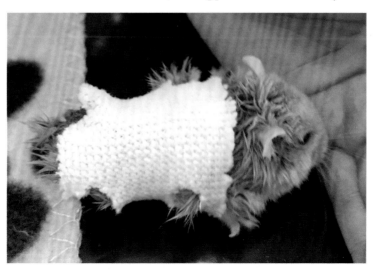

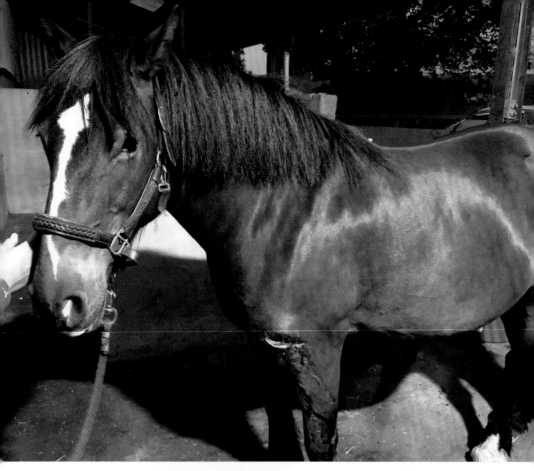

Kari, the horse down the strath, who managed to wound her leg quite seriously as shown here

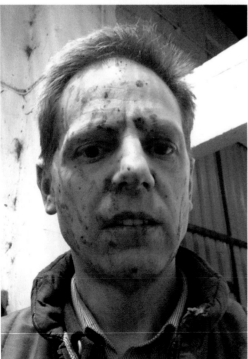

It was all going well until the cow I was operating on coughed!

SOME LESS USUAL CUSTOMERS

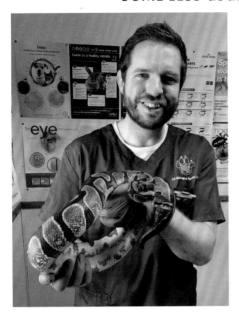

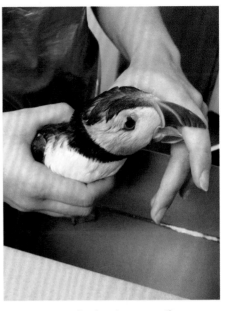

Vet Ken with a python

Learning the hard way. Puffins are not as cute as they look!

We have been known to treat the occasional swan too

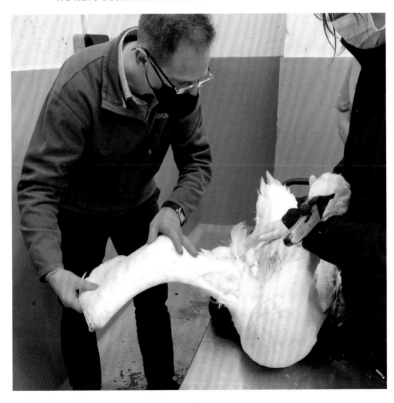

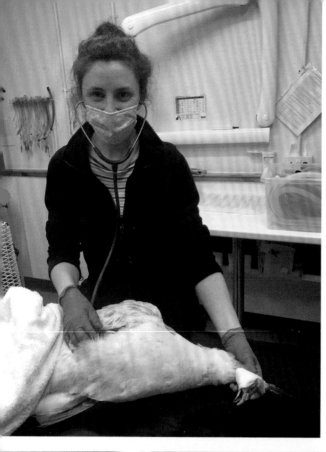

Vet Katie and I operated on the peahen that had previously appeared in an episode of *The Highland Vet*

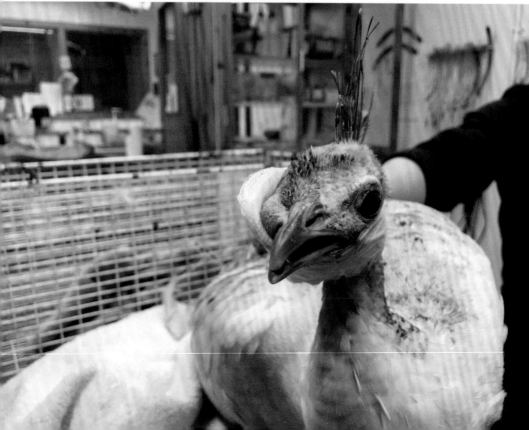

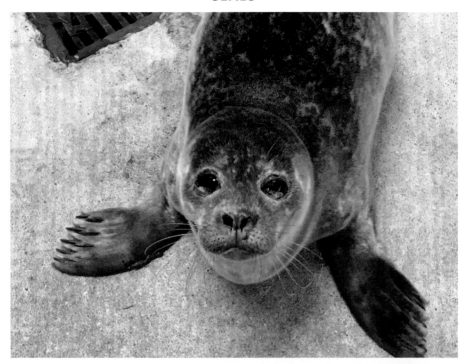

A harbour seal pup
who needed assistance
at the surgery in
December 2021.
Here vet William and
nurse Caitlin help to
administer oral fluids

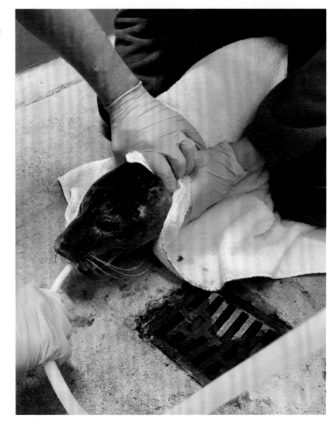

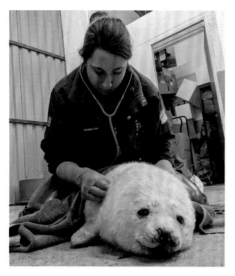

Vet Shondie with Pudding, the abandoned seal pup who featured on *The Highland Vet*

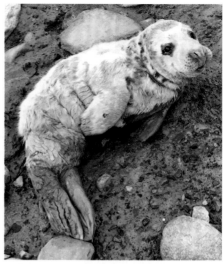

A lone seal pup I came across at the beach recently. There was a good chance its mother was coming back for it. I notified the SSPCA, who will hopefully have monitored the situation

LIGHT RELIEF

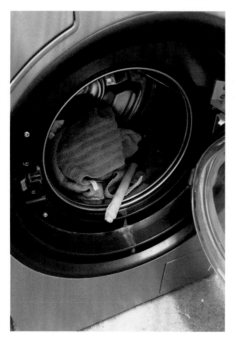

The 'leak' in the washing machine. Happily, the practice team have a good sense of humour

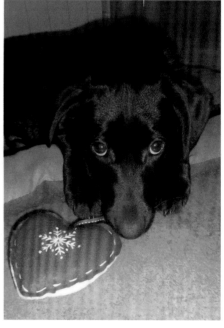

Our black lab Milis on Valentine's Day

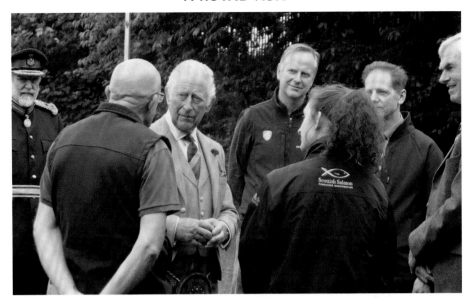

Lord Thurso and the Prince of Wales with vets William,
Iain, Katie, myself and retired vet Frank

The Prince of Wales's visit to the surgery in 2021.
Milis received a royal pat on the head!

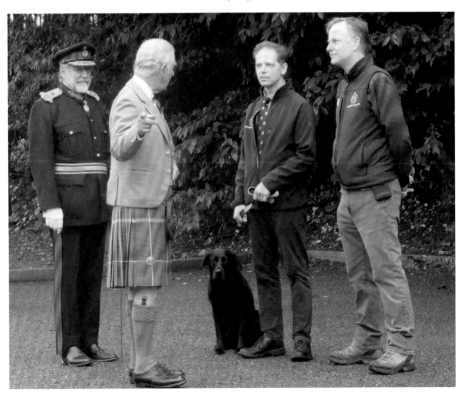

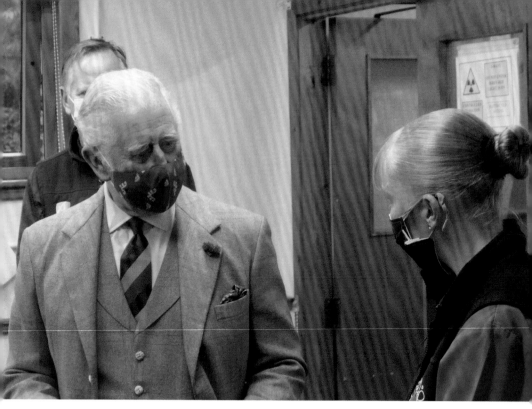

The Prince of Wales chatting with nurse Vicky, then meeting vet David's dog Bailey with nurse Caitlin and vets Eilidh and Iain

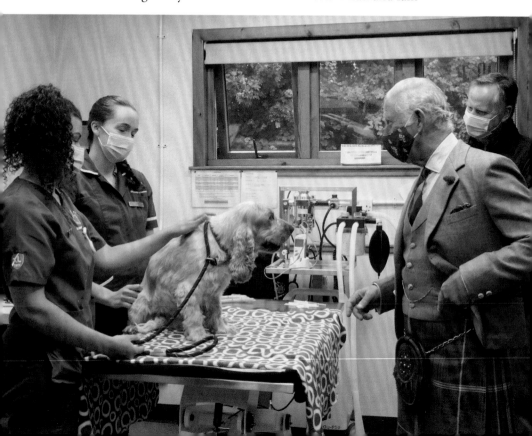

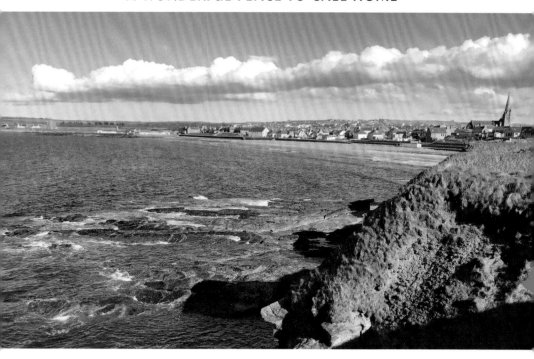

Thurso in the sun
and a typical Sutherland vista

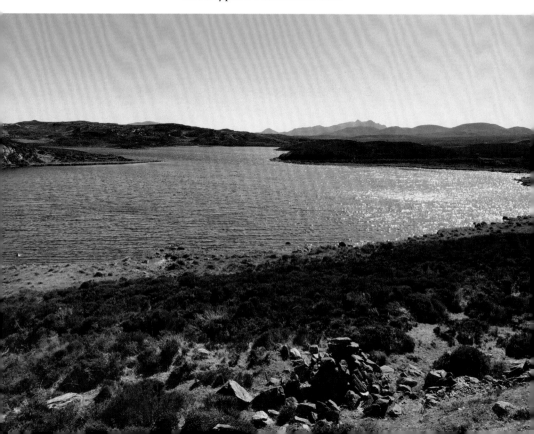

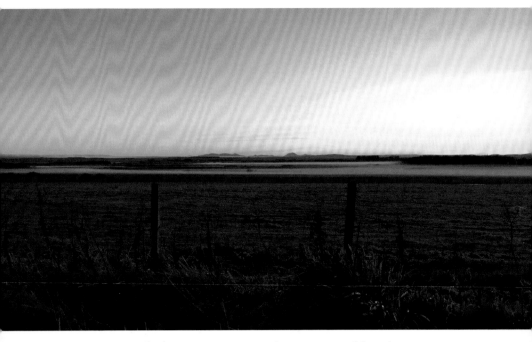

The late summer sunsets here are something else

Note the shining lighthouse on Dunnet Head at the far left of this image

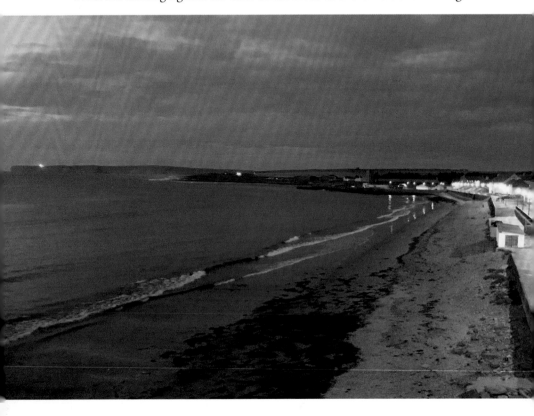

respite. He possibly had figures to push around for the business, although not perhaps before he'd indulged himself with a trip to buy a newspaper.

As other vets were leaving to attend their allotted calls, the phone rang. A receptionist told the only available vet that a farmer was wanting a cow to be cleaned. It could have been written directly in the diary as a call, but Frank said, 'I'll speak to him.' He lifted the receiver and sat down on the chair in the practice's kitchen.

From the adjacent office, I overheard the short discussion that followed. It was obvious Frank was not going to give up his call-free morning without good reason. He could not see the incredulous expression on my face as his broad Aberdonian voice affirmed with a reassuring tone, 'Dinnae worry, George, she'll be fine. Modern thinking is that cows don't need to be cleaned.'

As I said, change can filter slowly into our working practice. However, when necessary, it can be ushered in much more rapidly.

Summer

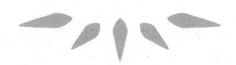

Chapter Thirteen

Let There Be Light!

In the lands stretching southwards away from the northern Highlands, a 'good' summer might often be judged by how hot it gets. Up here, though, we know we will never get those deep-orange splats that you see on the television weather forecasts, usually telling of a 30-degree heatwave somewhere in southern England.

At this latitude, if it passes 20 degrees, then that's considered to be a hot day, and such a temperature is ideal for working or wandering outdoors without wilting in the heat. I can't say I really envy those places that get high twenties or early thirties regularly. For me, the burning intensity of the light takes a poor second place to the quality and, moreover, sheer quantity of light we experience throughout our summers. Daylight, as it emerges from a long period of wintry repression, is something I try not to take for granted.

Because our planet is tilted on its axis, the further north you are situated, the greater number of daylight hours you will gradually receive during the northern hemisphere's summer, until you hit a peak at midsummer's longest day: the summer solstice in late

June. Indeed, in summer, the North Pole becomes the 'land of the midnight sun'. Come winter, though, the reverse is true, and for us in the far north, the sun will make only a brief appearance above the horizon each day around the winter solstice at Christmastime.

It really does take all that darkness to make you fully appreciate the daylight. In the height of summer, you can wake up as early as 4am and start to see the sun creeping into the sky. At that time of year, it won't get fully dark in the night at all; instead, you'll witness a beautiful inky gloaming: a twilight sky that shifts through darkened hues of blues and bruisy purples as the sun merely bobs below the horizon, ready to resurface bright and early.

It is slightly amusing to think that once the spring workload no longer disturbs your nights, the sun shows itself earlier and earlier, streaming through the window to continue to curtail your slumber! However, I refuse to grumble, but rather, make the most of this time of year. We have blackout blinds in our bedroom, which reduce sleep loss before we arise, and yet, on many summer nights I'll go to bed and deliberately leave a blind open, just for a few minutes. I then sit up in bed and look out across the sea to the craggy toe of land that forms the peninsula of Dunnet Head. Backlit by the dim glow of the sky beyond, the silhouette of this impressive promontory emits comforting, mesmerising bursts of illumination. The lighthouse, perched on top of a 300-foot-high weather-beaten clifftop for almost 200 years, is still pulsing out life-saving light across the Pentland Firth. On a calm summer's night, it is reassuring to consider the constancy of this beacon, faithful and unfailing throughout the storms and seasons.

In the colder months it can be a real challenge to motivate yourself to just get out of the door and go for a walk. You always feel the benefit afterwards, when you're back home sipping a mug of tea; but when the wind and rain are battering our coastline, and it's already pitch-black come dinnertime, slipping the lead onto the dog and heading out can feel like the opening to some Captain Scott-esque Antarctic tragedy: 'Jennifer, we are going out for a walk, and we may be some time.'

Come summer, though, by complete contrast, the warm calm of the late evening is enticing. As bedtime approaches, Jennifer or I will often look out of the window and suggest a stroll along the local beach or the clifftop. It is all too easy to lose a sense of the hour, you can be fooled into believing it's 8pm when in reality midnight is approaching. Your body clock is duped, and it can be hard to persuade yourself it's bedtime – and we need no more reasons for sleep deprivation!

There's another, subtler, quality to high summer in the middle of the night: the incredible stillness and quiet. I can remember driving home late from a farm job one summer's eve when I was suddenly taken with an urge to stop the car and get out. I was out in open country and, as I switched off the engine, climbed out into the warm air and allowed my senses to settle, I became acutely aware of a near-total silence. I was under the giant Caithness sky with an almost breathless breeze, listening to a captivating, dreamy, yet stunning quiet.

It was a moment to savour. I am as guilty as any of you for filling my life with noise – not just radio, TV, phones, internet, other people, but the ceaseless bustling within my own head. Indeed, some might fear that truly natural quiet is no longer available to us in modern-day Britain, yet here I was, with an ethereal stillness all around me, and it was free of charge. I may have been working late, but I felt an odd sense of privilege.

With the hard work of spring at least doubling the heads of cattle and sheep, the area is brimming with livestock. Without them, the counties in late spring and early summer would present a hugely disillusioning picture. With the sun on their backs and blue skies above, it is a deeply comforting scene, and the finest visual representation of quite how important farming is to the region.

It is a recognised cliché that lambs frolic in the fields, but adolescent calves do that too. In doing so, they shift a bulk some ten times that of a lamb and are thus somewhat more cumbersome. Both lambs and calves really pile on the pounds from birth, and within a few weeks they are nearly unrecognisable from those small, dazed, slime-covered parcels of fur that first staggered in the straw.

The young animals of early summer may look a lot older to the layman's eye, but they are still youngsters, and, particularly if the weather takes a nosedive, we can get a wave of sick infant animals requiring our attention. Parasites will also build up on pasture, adding their own spanner into the works. Or perhaps the fun and frolics of inexperienced youngstock will lead to straightforward accidents: limbs trapped in feed boxes or fences, or a juvenile coming off second-best from an encounter with the farmyard machinery. But sometimes an injury can also be due to the inexperience of the parent.

This year vet Rebecca treated a Zwartbles-cross lamb that required a splint because it was dragging its hind leg behind it as it walked. The plausible cause of the injury? Its mum had accidentally sat on it sometime during the night. Another example of a more unusual parental calamity came in the second season of *The Highland Vet*, where farmer George arrived at the surgery with a three-week-old calf with its nose very badly wounded.

It is perfectly normal maternal behaviour for a cow or sheep to lick a newborn clean of all the fluid, mucus and placental membranes coating the body after birth. Indeed, when it comes to the face, especially the baby's nose and mouth, it can be an important step in reducing the chances of it suffocating. This poor calf, though, had lost almost its entire nose to its mum's obsessive over-diligence.

The tongue of an adult cow is rough to the touch, almost like light sandpaper, so, with repeated licking, this mum had done some real damage to her charge. This was a first for both us as vets and the farmer and required immediate surgery to close the wound.

Occasionally, it is an apparent lack of maternalism that can cause problems. We do actually have cases where calves are quite badly beaten up by their own mothers. They might pick them up and throw them to the other side of a pen, headbutt them or even kick them.

It is difficult to know exactly what is going through the mind of the mother in those cases. A bit of maternal vigour to physically stimulate the calf immediately after birth is normal, just to goad it into action if it is struggling to breathe or stand. A more violent beating could be an excessive extension of such behaviour, or it might just be that the mum simply hasn't yet bonded with her offspring and wants to keep them well away. Additionally, a mother kicking a calf to prevent suckling may be down to something as simple as a sore udder.

A calf might be attacked by another cow too, perhaps if the wee thing mistakes her milk supply for its mother's. But whatever the cause, heavyweight adult animals can do an awful lot of damage to the young: broken limbs, deep bruising, internal bleeding or big open wounds. We have to fix them up as best we can, but it is then ultimately down to the farmer to find solutions to keep the young animals as safe as possible, at least until they have become more robust and worldly wise, or their mothers have relaxed to a less aggressive frame of mind.

It is a harsh reality experienced by a minority of lambs and calves, but, sadly, sometimes life in the world of animals can be very cruel.

Chapter Fourteen

Cats, Dogs, and Saying Goodbye

I've kept pets for almost all of my life.

I had guinea pigs as a boy, which saw me take the classic animal-keeping journey of many children: an interest in the creatures themselves but less of an enthusiasm for tending to them and cleaning them out! But, fortunately (I say only with mature hindsight), I had parents who instilled a sense of responsibility in their kids. However, mostly our house kept to the traditional route of cat and dog ownership.

We had Pepsi, a springer spaniel, who was very much part of the household and typical for her breed: weeing when excited to see us and running off after smells. We also had many an extra 'dog walk' on account of the garden gate having been accidentally left open, which would result in us searching both street and field to locate her. 'Claws' was tabby and white, a typical loner of a cat who did his own thing out and about, so my memories of him are few. I recall we got him around Christmastime, because we had relatives staying. I can picture the kitten crawling along my dad's legs as he reclined on the sofa, only for one of my cheeky cousins to quip, 'He's getting close to the danger zone', suggesting the curious feline wouldn't make it to adulthood if he ventured too close to my dad's stinky feet.

There are some strong, often humorous, stereotypes of dogs, cats and the differences between them as pets. *You choose to own a dog, but a cat chooses you* might resonate with some pet owners. Fickle felines will happily move into a house across the road if they find the company, food and cosy furniture more to their liking. It is true each species often seems to play its expected role, but, as with most stereotypes, there is always room for a fair bit of mould breaking. Take these common misconceptions, for example:

Cats look after their own exercise and toilet habits, whereas dogs need walks and poop-scoops. Yet, a dog with a huge garden and a dog flap would function pretty much like a cat, although it's always nice to get out for wider exploration elsewhere. It is perhaps more a case of a difference in the human keeping the pet. A dog or cat will both be kept as our companions, but we keep dogs because we want to get out in the fresh air with them. Then, of course, there are the cats who have the whole of the outdoors as their latrine (yes, even next door's flower beds) but, instead, must come inside for a private poo in the litter box. Rather pongy and hardly low-maintenance!

Cats eat what they need, but dogs will gorge until they pop is another rule of thumb. I've heard that the majority of cats will moderate their own food intake (and thus body weight) in the face of ad-lib provision, yet many rather rotund individuals prove this is most definitely not a 100 per cent rule. On the other hand, there are a few well-tempered canines who eat just what they need and no more – although, true, most would eat what they can, as quickly as they can. This is actually a very useful veterinary yardstick; a diminished appetite is a good indication that all is not well.

Dogs demand more company. Cats are solitary and aloof, coming to you on their terms. Again, perhaps a fair generalisation, but have you met the cats who just won't leave you alone? You sit down – they are there on your lap. Working at your computer? They're dancing on the keys, obscuring your view. You leave the room – incessant meowing issues from behind the closed door.

The first dog I actually owned as an adult was a rescued golden retriever. It was in the years before Thurso, or having children of our own, when the Scottish Society for the Prevention of Cruelty to Animals (SSPCA) brought a three-to-four-month-old puppy into the surgery I was working at, down in Perth. She had been found abandoned by the roadside with a suspected broken jaw; however, on examination, I deduced that the jaw fracture was actually quite old, and her jawline had since permanently set in a slightly wonky position.

Luckily, she wasn't in any pain, and, that night, I took her home to our little cottage just outside the city. It was my birthday that day, so I knew I had some leverage should I need it (I very well might have done, given the first thing she did on entry to our home was poo all over the rug), but I needn't have worried. Jennifer took to her instantly (I cleaned up the poo!) and we ended up adopting her as our own, naming her Fyrish, after a notable hill topped with a monument near Jennifer's childhood home.

Our next dog, Poppy, came off the back of an entirely sleepless night of work in the calving season here in Thurso. It was about

10pm when I was called out to the surgery to take a look at a yellow Labrador that was going into labour. I examined her and concluded that she was some way off delivery. I suggested we give her an hour or so, and, in the interim, I was called to a tricky calving on one of our farms. On my return to the surgery I called the Lab's owner. There had been no progress, and so, in the small hours of the morning, I took the decision to conduct a caesarean section.

The mother had a lovely nature and I had really started to warm to her. Despite being in a stressful situation, she'd remained very calm and compliant.

A little before dawn, I delivered her litter of pups, a mix of boys and girls but all black, her own colouring dominated by the father's genetics. I asked if they all had prospective owners. 'I might actually be quite interested in taking one, perhaps the smallest female in the litter.' The voice of reason in my head lost the battle to my sleep-deprived consciousness.

It was just a passing comment, really, but I was serious enough to test the water with Jennifer about it when I finally returned home for breakfast. We had missed having a dog around since we'd had to say goodbye to Fyrish earlier that year, and the children had only known a grown dog, never a puppy.

A couple of days later, I rang the owner. 'I'm not sure if you can remember, but I mentioned that I might be interested in having one of the pups. Is that still okay?' I discovered that my vague, non-committal comment on the night of the operation had been assumed a done deal: 'The little girl is all yours.' And that was how Poppy became another four-legged addition to our family.

Fyrish was not the only rescue to come into our house. Before her, we had already rescued two cats.

It was my first week working as a newly qualified vet, in what was my first job in a general practice. Jennifer was naturally quite keen to come and have a look around. Late one evening, I was on call and offered to show her around the surgery – the public area, the operating theatre, the consulting rooms. As we entered the kennel room, a single patient peered at us through the metal bars. I opened the cage and scooped a cute little ginger-and-white kitten into Jennifer's arms, its badly damaged tail all too obvious. I explained that he was homeless and so, unless someone wanted to take him on as a going concern, he was destined for euthanasia.

Jennifer looked distraught. 'Well,' I attempted in comfort, 'I could operate on his tail myself tomorrow and then bring him home to ours?'

I am in no doubt that Jennifer saw right through my very deliberate ploy. What could she say, really?! I amputated the tail and that was that: Splat was ours. Yes, sorry, on considering the state of his tail, my unfortunate sense of humour led us to an obvious name.

Splat was a bit of a mad cat. His need for affection seemed to vary from demanding it was showered upon him, to being totally dismissive of us, but his oddest quirk was that he really liked to eat grass. It's not utterly unheard of. Non-grass-eating animals will sometimes eat grass if they have a sore stomach and want to make themselves sick; but, in the absence of any obvious clinical explanation to his owner-cum-vet, Splat did it completely out of habit, and seemed to actively enjoy it. He also liked to feast on daddy-long-legs, filling his stomach with them in the summer before vomiting them back up onto the kitchen floor.

In spite of his peculiarities and his troubled start to life, I'm pleased to say good old Splat lived to a ripe old age with us and was greatly missed when he eventually passed away.

It's fair to say, the names of our cats don't inhabit anything like the same level of romance and forethought as our dogs. That's not to say we cared for them any less. It's just, I suppose, we were a bit more matter-of-fact with their names. After explaining how Splat was named, I'm actually a little embarrassed to set in type the name of cat number two, so I'll give you the background first and hope for your forgiveness later!

He was another rescue, this time an abandoned newborn kitten. Newborns need regular feeding, so I took him home with me and got up to feed him in the middle of the night with a small modified syringe filled with milk formula. It was never our intention to keep him; we just thought we'd get him through the early stage of his life and then find appropriate new owners, so we didn't give him a name per se. Instead (okay, here comes the embarrassing bit), we'd just say to each other, 'Have you fed the little git yet?'

'Git' grew well and soon endeared himself to his surrogate parents, so we decided it was best that we just keep him. However, despite our efforts to work with other, more reasonable, names beginning with 'G', unfortunately, his (I promise!) affectionate nickname stuck for the rest of his days.

Clearly, it wasn't a name we'd given too much attention to, and, unlike a dog, it wasn't as if we were going to be shouting it out loud in a public place anyway. As a 'pre-child' couple at that time, what we hadn't really thought through was that pets would be an obvious topic for projects and classroom discussions when our girls entered primary school. For them, our household animals had simply always 'been'. I shudder to think what went through the minds of their teachers when, in all innocence, they proudly proclaimed 'Splat and Git' as their beloved cats.

I can imagine the dumbfounded faces and stifled chuckles. 'But, hold on, isn't your dad the local vet?'

Virtually all of the vets and staff in our practice have pets. That should hardly be a surprise in itself; to pursue this profession, you are almost certain to be an animal lover. But as a vet, owning a pet does also give you the requisite empathy to imagine yourself in the shoes of those whose sick or injured animals you are responsible for.

I would guess, in any profession that has an element of 'care' – whether that be in human or veterinary medicine, or working with the disabled, the elderly, or people with mental health problems – just having that direct personal experience can make a real difference. I feel it helps make us more plausible when offering advice and opinions. And I sincerely hope we can be a real source of comfort and reassurance at times of emotional trauma, such as in the situation of having to put to sleep a much-loved pet.

I've lost dogs and cats that are very dear to me. I know exactly how horrible it feels when you have to face losing an animal that is, and has been for so long, central to your life and home. The truth is, despite knowing full well that the shorter lifespan of an animal means that you'll probably lose several during your lifetime, there is still no easy way to say goodbye.

Of course, some passings aren't quite as hard as others. I remember with Git, it all started with a sudden behavioural change. Despite being hand-reared at birth, he turned out to be quite a, well, anti-social little git! He would crawl under the bed, hide behind the washing machine, go outside all day long, and generally keep himself to himself. Then one day he suddenly came through to where Jennifer and I were sat and just wanted attention: to be petted and stroked, to be close. We soon realised he was gravely ill and, within 24 hours, he was gone. It was heartwarming that he sought our company in those final hours.

From our perspective as vets, when it comes to putting an animal down, we try to make the process as smooth and painless as it can possibly be. These are the times when a perfect blend of clinical and people skills becomes paramount. Being practical and slick with the procedure might seem superficially unemotional, but believe me, it really matters to animal and owner, and allows you the space to fully engage with the emotions and feelings in the room.

You also need to allow the owner space to deal with it all in their own way. Some are quiet and require just brief reassurances from the vet, while others process it externally, telling you all about their pet's quirks and personality and numerous stories from their lives. A box of tissues, a sympathetic ear and enough time set aside to avoid a sense of rush are essential.

One of our cats was put down by another vet, and the other was put to sleep by me; but I wasn't present for either Fyrish's or Poppy's passing. With Poppy, it was physically impossible for me to be present, but with Fyrish, I just couldn't face it. I asked my colleagues to attend to it, and Frank kindly paid a visit to our house while I distracted myself with work. With Jennifer present, he gave Fyrish a painless injection to help her slip away.

The circumstances of Poppy's passing were extremely hard, though, for more than just our family. We were all on holiday in France with friends when Poppy suddenly fell very ill. She'd had a bit of diarrhoea before we'd left, but that was nothing unusual for a Lab that scavenges by the river; I presumed it would settle down quickly, as such things normally do. Eileen, one of our receptionists, was looking after her, and we headed off on holiday without feeling too concerned.

A couple of days later, though, Eileen warned me that Poppy wasn't getting any better; in fact, she was a whole lot worse. The surgery leapt into action: all the tests were run and I soon received an emailed scan of Poppy's abdomen. A kidney looked enlarged. Some form of surgery would be required.

There were three options on the table: the quickest was to let my colleagues take on the surgery themselves, with my permission; alternatively, Poppy could have been referred to a specialist; or, finally, I could fly home and deal with her myself.

Poppy was young – she hadn't even turned eight – and as far as I was concerned, the decision was very straightforward. I trusted the team. I knew they were fantastic vets, I had every confidence in them and I was certain they would do all they could. I felt bad leaving Eileen and my clinical colleagues with all the pressure and responsibility, but I also felt there was nothing to be gained from a referral, and me coming back wasn't going to make a difference to Poppy's quality of care, and would certainly cause a delay. If it were truly as serious as it looked, they needed to get into her abdomen right away, and Poppy was either going to make it or she wasn't.

As my family and friends walked in the sunshine along a French riverbank, a surgical team began the operation back home in Thurso. I kept the news from the children, not wanting to cause worry on something we no longer had any control over. I was hoping for the best, when my mobile phone started to ring. My family rolled their eyes, thinking, *The practice won't leave Dad alone even when he's in another country!* I didn't set them straight.

Bridget and Ken had indeed discovered a huge abnormal kidney inside Poppy. I asked them to try to remove it, but it was futile; it was crumbling in their fingers and the blood loss was scary. Ken called again to tell me that they hadn't been able to save her. I requested he send a sample for pathological analysis. On my return, the report was waiting for me: it had all been in vain – Poppy had had a nasty cancer.

By the French riverside, I hung up the phone and looked over to my girls, all having fun and laughing with our friends. Jennifer and I kept it to ourselves for the day, but that evening we took them out for a walk and I broke the news. I can still picture their faces in my mind. The tears flowed and flowed.

Even as a vet who knows the practical realism of animal ownership inside out, recalling how I felt then has given me an awful lot of time for people as they say goodbye. It can be absolutely heartbreaking.

Chapter Fifteen

Of Lost Dogs and Jellyfish

Our latest dog is called Milis (pronounced 'Meelish'). The name is Gaelic for 'sweet' and was the nickname given to my father-in-law by his mother when he was a boy. Milis came to us somewhat undramatically by way of my wife's hairdresser – although, thematically, it was my birthday again. One of the things that had become obvious to us in the build-up to getting her was, quite honestly, just how little we were getting out for daily walks since our dear Poppy had passed on.

Despite your best intentions, it is pretty amazing how quickly you find yourself making excuses to not get out for a walk when you don't have the responsibility of exercising a dog – especially when the weather is truly foul. And not doing so meant we were not only missing out on fresh air and exercise, but we had also stopped exploring all the places a dog can take you to.

Up here in summer, not getting outside should be a borderline criminal act; but as much as taking your four-legged friend into the great outdoors is one of the real pleasures of owning a dog, it does come with the occasional side serving of very real stress.

Come June in Caithness and north Sutherland, we will have already welcomed a steady flow of tourists, all keen to experience the natural beauty of these northern counties for themselves.

If you had never visited, and were just presented with an image of one of our local beaches, you could be forgiven for thinking you were looking at a patch of coast somewhere in the South Pacific and not, in fact, the Highlands of Scotland.

We really are spoilt. Some of our beaches stretch out as dazzling arcs of appealing golden sand. Others have wave-rounded pebbles and inviting rock pools. Nearly all are backdropped by immense sand dunes or weathered sandstone cliffs with towering sea stacks and arches. If you were to transplant our entire coastline to the south of England, I am sure it would very quickly become choked with people.

But our remoteness works in our favour; tourism up here has to be a very deliberate act and not a spur-of-the-moment day trip. We do see a noticeable seasonal rise in holiday traffic and busyness on the beaches, but, for now at least, the footfall here is such that you'll always have plenty of room; and, off-peak on a clear winter's day, you may even have an entire stunning beach to yourself.

I almost feel a little conflicted in telling the whole truth about just how beautiful the north coast beaches really are, lest they all become the 'Costa del Scotland' overnight, but I think another big factor in deterring the sun worshippers is that our average temperature and frequent breeze leave few days each year where the beach is suitable for bathing suits and bronzing. However, that makes those days all the more special when they occur; Thurso's beach and esplanade look like the Spanish Riviera for a brief afternoon, and if we're lucky, Ken will appear back from a call with ice creams for all.

Open-water swimming seems to have become popular whatever the season, but as alluring as those crystalline azure waters may often look in midsummer, I have only ever been drawn to submerse myself in their salty depths on one occasion, and can definitely confirm that the sea is as heart-stoppingly cold as you might expect for northern Scotland! Surfing is a major activity up here, but at least surfers have the sense to wear wetsuits.

For many British dog owners, one of the joys of a domestic holiday is being able to take your four-legged friend with you. The North Coast 500 launched officially in 2015. This is a 516-mile road route around much of the Highland's coastline, which existed long before it was given a name, but since then we have seen a steady growth in the popularity of Caithness and Sutherland as a tourist destination. Inevitably, this means that there are increasing occasions when dog-loving holidaymakers will be forced to engage with our services.

Usually, they will have phoned in advance before bringing their dog in, which at least allows us to arrange for a clinical history of the animal to be emailed from their vets back home, prior to their arrival. Obviously, though, there are plenty of medical cases where, if we can't get hold of such records quickly, we can work without them, especially if we're dealing with a case of a random injury or accident.

Any dog can have a misadventure, and in the summer on our beaches there are cases each year where dogs have made the mistake of getting a little too intimately acquainted with our local population of jellyfish. Luckily, none of our jellyfish are particularly dangerous or excruciatingly painful (unless you have an adverse allergic reaction) – at least not on the scale of, say, Australia's lethal box jellyfish; but any jellyfish sting is nonetheless very uncomfortable.

Jellyfish are regularly encountered washed up and beached below the high tideline, or just hovering around in the paddle zone. Dogs are naturally quite curious animals, and, unfortunately, the way they engage with the world is all too frequently with their nose, tongue and mouth – none of which I would recommend as particularly sensible areas of one's anatomy for safe jellyfish exploration.

Discomfort is inescapable as hundreds of microscopic barbed stingers called nematocysts stab into the dog's body, and the swallowing of a tentacle will frequently cause dogs to drool and vomit. Understandably, their owners will then become quite worried at seeing such an apparently adverse reaction. However, after the vomiting and salivation subside, the dog has usually simply learnt a useful lesson about what not to investigate on a fine summer's day at the beach; I am yet to see a dog come to serious harm from engaging with jellyfish.

Vet William advocates a drink of milk to soothe the mouth and oesophagus. Vinegar is supposed to help neutralise the stingy nematocysts, but dousing a dog's mouth with vinegar is likely to elicit a reaction similar to that which the jellyfish has already caused! If they are brought into us, we might give them a medication to reduce the pain and their feeling of queasiness before reassuring the owner that, as violent as the short-term reaction to a jellyfish seems, it is highly unlikely to be fatal, at least in Scotland.

That's not to say there aren't some real summer dangers for dogs when they explore wet environments. Blue-green algae is something that has generated some grave headlines in recent years, particularly with the upturns in hot summer weather as our climate changes.

It is not something we encounter with real regularity up here due to our more moderate summers, but blue-green algae has been found in Caithness's Loch Watten in the last couple of years, and it is becoming much more prevalent further south in Scotland, with particularly nasty blooms breaking out on Loch Lomond this summer.

The algae itself is naturally occurring and sun-loving, and tends to form in very obvious vivid-green or, not surprisingly, blue-green patches around the edges of still water, especially where there is a high concentration of organic matter. For humans, contact with these algae can cause skin irritation and sickness, but for livestock, waterbirds, fish and dogs, it is potentially deadly.

Walking along the banks of a loch or river on a hot summer's day, I'm sure most dog owners would think very little of allowing their animal into the water for a quick drink or swim, but therein lies the danger. The algae itself is technically a type of bacteria called cyanobacteria, and although not all blue-green algal blooms are dangerous, some do produce toxins that are extremely harmful, particularly to a dog's nervous system and liver. Fatalities can occur scarily rapidly, even within 15 minutes of ingestion. Dogs can take it in either by drinking it directly or by licking it off their coats after a swim.

Most areas prone to blue-green algae will have clear signage and warnings whenever it is present, but nonetheless, if you spot any such algae, keep your dog well away from it. Sadly, there is no antidote to algae poisoning at present, but the treatment is remarkably similar to that of Jess the cat, who took the poisonous lily pollen. We can give a dog an emetic drug to make it sick, activated charcoal to absorb the toxins, and intensive intravenous fluid therapy, along with other supportive treatments if the dog is fitting or struggling to breathe.

Holidaymakers, and locals, do occasionally manage to lose their dogs – or rather, dogs take themselves off for a wee wander. I'm sure the vast majority of dog owners have been there at some point. I know I certainly have. Most dogs, even those that are thoroughly well trained, can be lured away at times. Plainly put: if a dog sees or smells something exceptionally enticing, then you, and whatever treats you are carrying, become dull and uninteresting by comparison. They'll shoot off after that rabbit, deer or whiff of rotting carcass a mile upwind, and there isn't a whole lot you can do about it.

People don't lose their dogs only on walks, though. I've lost my dogs on more than a couple of occasions after they somehow managed to escape our gated garden and take themselves off for a stroll. And I know there are plenty of people who have unknowingly left a door or gate ajar, only for a wet nose and paw to later exploit the opportunity.

Reuniting lost dogs with their owners is something we will do as a free service to the community. It's not really one of our official roles, but, inevitably, when people don't know where to turn, having either lost or found a dog, they think, *Let's try the vet's.* We have a microchip scanner in the surgery, which, whenever a dog is discovered and brought in to us, we can then use to find the owner's details and make contact (as long as the animal has been chipped).

There is a much easier, more traditional, way of reuniting a dog, and possibly even a cat, with a fretting owner. Don't overlook the far more readily useful engraved disc that you can simply and cheaply place on your animal's collar. By just putting your contact details on there, you are likely to get your cat or dog back more rapidly than by invoking the whole rigmarole of them coming to us, or another establishment, to be scanned. The microchips are useful for contest of ownership, and, of course, as a failsafe if the little disc is missing or the details have rubbed off over time; but in my opinion, the simplest methods are so often the best. In this day and age, where everyone carries a mobile phone in their pocket, a finder can call you directly using the number on the tag. Why make someone who finds your dog somewhere out in the countryside travel miles into town to get it scanned, only for them to discover that you are out there, not far from where they were, looking for your dog!

I had an amusing lost dog incident this summer. A member of the public turned up at our surgery with a Yorkshire terrier they had found, which we duly scanned before calling up the owner. So far: so straightforward. However, despite a few efforts at calling, we just couldn't get hold of the listed owner. Usually, that's not so much of a problem, as frequently we are among the first ports of call when someone realises that they've lost a pet. This time, though, the hours ticked by and we received no call.

Luckily, thanks to the microchip, we not only had the owner's number, we had the dog's name and address too. The owner had five Yorkies and she lived in town, so I decided to pop past in person. I couldn't work out exactly where the front door to the house was so I knocked on a window, which unleashed the yapping of many small canine mouths. It was impossible to see into the garden due to a high wall and a tall, solid wooden gate, but the yapping migrated towards the gate, and then it opened.

'Have you lost a Yorkie?' I began.

The grey-haired lady looked bemused, even indignant. She glanced around her feet at the swarm of Yorkies. 'No,' she replied confidently, despite the fact we'd had a dog listed as hers in our surgery for a good five hours by that point.

'Well,' I asked, 'what about Douglas?'

Her face suddenly became concerned, given she definitely *did* own a dog by that name and was clearly surprised that I was being so specific.

She studied the pack of pooches at her ankles, before looking up, slightly red-faced. 'Oh! You're right! I have lost wee Douglas!' When you have so many small creatures darting here and there, could she really be blamed for thinking that four were still five? She had spent the day aware of a different Yorkie or two out of the corner of each eye, so why would she imagine they weren't all present?

It was all very good-natured, and a happy reunion ensued. I didn't rub it in; we too, had once had a dog of ours returned to us before we'd even realised it was missing, and we only had one!

One of the most dramatic lost dog stories in my career happened a good few years ago now. I was called out by a fisherman who had discovered a dog down on the riverbank some distance out of town. He said, over the phone, that it was a yellow Labrador and was in quite some state: lethargic, thin and curled up in the river-side reeds as if it were about to die.

I went down to the location with a nurse. We parked up and walked across two fields and then along the riverside, over quite rough terrain, in search of this unfortunate animal. We eventually found it among the vegetation and, true to the angler's word, it really was in desperate trouble. In fact, it was so emaciated and weak, it was incapable of standing up on its own legs.

I had to carry the Labrador all the way back to my car over uneven ground and across the fields; good job I was younger and fitter back then! Although, the job was made easier by the dog's skeletal form. I drove him straight to the surgery for emergency fluids, food and warmth.

When we scanned the chip, we discovered that the owner wasn't a local at all. My understanding was that they had come to Caithness for a short trip, lost the dog on a walk, and, after a great deal of searching, had eventually reached the point where they'd had little choice but to give up.

This was a time before the social media boom. Today, people can canvass the accounts of multiple local groups and businesses and soon have an army of people aware of their lost animal; but with this dog, as the weeks had elapsed, all hope of finding him alive had vanished.

I could scarcely believe how long this dog had been fending for himself down by the river: he had spent *weeks* in the wild. There was little wonder he had lost so much weight. The finding was timely – he was about to starve to death.

I assumed he had managed to scavenge some small amount of food on the banks at some point, and that he had been drinking the river water, but, as a domesticated animal, that was only ever going to get him so far. I felt it was quite an unusual situation:

I don't know why the dog, being a pet, hadn't behaved more as we might all guess, by seeking out humans, wandering into farmyards or along the river into town to find gardens and bins to raid.

As you can imagine, the owner was beyond ecstatic, and very shocked, to hear their dog had been found alive; no doubt the dog had all but given up hope of ever seeing them again too. But the story proved the value of a form of identification – be it a tag or microchip – as well as the enduring kindness of strangers, when it comes to rescuing animals in dire circumstances.

I touched on the danger of being in fields with cows and calves in the spring section. Real threat to your safety is the only scenario where you might consider dropping your dog's lead and making a dash for it. The rest of the time – and especially in late spring and summer, when there are so many young lambs in the fields – you should stick to the public footpaths and not allow your dog to run around off the lead in fields with any livestock, even if they seem to be very far away.

You may also enter a field thinking it is empty of animals, but there have been many times when I've been out walking the dog and livestock has appeared seemingly from nowhere, usually from a blind spot behind the brow of a hill. And then there's always the chance a farmer could unexpectantly open a gate and drive a whole herd of animals into where you're walking.

Vets and farmers have heard the assumptions of well-meaning owners that couldn't countenance the idea that their dog could ever harm another animal, but even so, it does happen, and many lambs and sheep die every year in Britain from dog attacks.

You can find yourself in serious trouble as an owner if your dog has killed a sheep. I remember working down in Perth many moons ago and having to make a dog sick in front of the police to determine whether it had sheep-attack evidence (wool, etc.) in its stomach. It is an all-round unpleasant and uncomfortable scenario. On one hand, you have an owner who may be facing the prospect of their dog being put down by a police order, as well as an expensive compensation payment to the sheep farmer; and on the other hand, you have the sheep farmer, who has just gone through the whole trial of spring only for their sheep to be horrifically hunted down and torn apart in the field.

It isn't just that dogs off the lead can kill sheep; sometimes they will simply maul them, frequently leaving them with severe lacerations and open wounds that we are then called in to stitch. And, during spring, the act of a dog simply chasing a heavily pregnant sheep around a field, without even laying paw or tooth on it, can be enough stress for it to suffer a miscarriage.

There are, of course, very legitimate reasons for certain breeds of dog to be off the lead and in the sheep fields. Working dogs, such as the iconic Border collie sheepdog, are trained from birth in the ability to manage and move sheep. The calls and whistles of the sheep farmer go hand in crook with the rearing and raising of sheepdogs, and, as the summer rolls forward, the sheep need to be gathered from the fields en masse to have their thick fleeces sheared from their bodies.

Where a pet dog exists for leisure and is an integral part of the family, a working dog is a professional in its own right and is an integral part of the team. Whether it's a sheepdog, a police dog or a guide dog, the training alone is a huge investment of time and, often, financial resources. That means you are only ever going to choose breeds that have both the temperament and mental capacity, in addition to the slick speed and agility, needed to execute those higher-level instructions. With sheepdogs, a proven bloodline can be of immense value. The offspring of champion sheepdogs could sell for the cost of a family car, especially if they have already received and responded to elite training. In 2021, the most expensive sheepdog of all time was confirmed at auction: £27,100 as the hammer dropped, for a 12-month-old collie.

A dog that can gather and move sheep across open fields and through narrow gates is a uniquely gifted creature, so the price is well worth paying. What it can also mean is that when a dog is injured or sick, it's the equivalent to a farm suddenly being without one of its most critical pieces of machinery.

The pressure to get that team member back on their feet, and back to work, as quickly as possible can weigh on the vet and farmer alike. There has been many a crestfallen sheep farmer in my time who, when I've explained that the broken bone or dislocated joint will leave their animal out of action for at least two months, still replies with a hopelessly desperate 'But I really need the dog now.'

The difference between a pet dog and a working dog is actually best demonstrated down on the farms themselves. Here you may well encounter a farmer who has perhaps two or three working collies, kept in their unheated kennels; they live an outdoor life, having been trained for a strict set of duties – focused, purposeful. And then there's the farmer's pet dog: a spoilt member of the leisure class that contributes absolutely nothing to the business, yet seemingly has its every whim and whine attended to, as if *they* were actually the most important creature in the county.

It is quite comical to behold really: a collie getting bossed around a field, toiling hard in all weathers and terrains; wearing its unkempt, dirt-matted coat almost as some sort of badge of honour. Compare this to the highly pampered pooch warming by the range in the farmhouse kitchen, fed choice titbits, groomed and mollycoddled. It's almost as if, in the farmer's mind, the two dogs are a separate species altogether.

I recall being arm-deep in a cow one day on one of our farms. The family of farmers, including the easy-going matriarch called Mary, were standing by, clad in wellies and waterproofs and chatting from the other side of the cattle crate. I hadn't noticed the strange subtle bulge in Mary's zipped-up oilskin jacket until it started wriggling. Had I entered a sci-fi twilight zone? Was she about to scream as an alien lifeform grotesquely burst from her body? No, just then, a small furry head appeared at the neckline of her jacket like a joey peeping from a kangaroo's pouch. A miniature poodle had been cosying in, being carried around the smelly farm where its pampered paws would most certainly not wish to be set down.

Sometimes a working dog can cross over the divide. We once treated a young working collie that had such a serious case of tetanus it very nearly died. It had a long, intensive stay at the surgery before being sent home for rehabilitation, and subsequently never left the comforts of the farmhouse again. Also, there are a handful of 'hybrids' out there: working collies that get to stay in the family home rather than in an outdoor kennel. For these dogs, this is definitely a case of having the best of both worlds.

However, the best example I ever saw of the contrasting sentiments harboured for farmyard canines actually came from a most unlikely-looking big softie.

Each summer, the Highland Games are held in Halkirk, Caithness. With bagpipes and kilts aplenty, it is a quintessentially Scottish affair. Established in 1886, the Games attract audiences in their thousands to watch people of all ages compete in activities such as traditional Highland dance, track and field events, cycling and clay pigeon shooting. Of course, the renowned tests of raw strength are a big draw for the crowds at Highland Games up and down the land. Although women also participate nowadays, it was traditionally the kilt-wearing strongmen who, for many, epitomised the gatherings. Mostly, these contests revolve around throwing very heavy things as far as possible: from the classic caber toss to the more mainstream shotput, and from the medieval-looking ball-and-chain and the hammer (a shaft of flexible cane attached to a weighted metal ball) right through to the unusual 'sheaf': a 16lb bag filled with grass, hand-hurled using a pitchfork. Tartan, testosterone, sweat and solid muscle: a veritable Scottish spectacle.

One of the farms in our patch is worked by a family of brothers, at least a couple of whom were strong and fierce competitors in the Halkirk Games. You could not miss these boys, built for purpose: solid beer-barrel chests, backs wide enough to land a jumbo jet upon, and biceps bigger than my waist. For the rest of the year, in overalls rather than a kilt, it is a physique greatly beneficial for coping with the rigors of hard graft on the farm.

Murdo, one of the brothers, had a red boxer that stuck to him like glue. Though he was pragmatic regarding the many head of cattle he tended, it was nevertheless clear that Murdo's sentiments ran much deeper for Milly; he adored his canine companion and doted upon her. Too big to fit kangaroo-style under a jacket, she broke the mould slightly and, despite snoozing in farmhouse comfort, enjoyed full run of the farm, paws in poo – the works.

Murdo's family shared a sizeable farm, so our visits were common enough. Several vets on several visits over the last few months had been pulled aside, after they'd completed whatever livestock task they had been performing, to inspect the leg of the beloved dog. Milly had developed a lump on a lower foreleg that had been gradually expanding in size. I had not been one of those vets, but I entered play when, one Saturday morning, Murdo appeared at the counter in the surgery to pick up some medication and spied me through the window.

He showed me a photo of the lumpy leg on his phone. The sad truth was that the lump wasn't simply large; such a mass on a lower limb made it a real problem from a surgical perspective. One by one, the vets he'd asked had all suggested it could well be inoperable, unless he were to consider amputation; so perhaps it was best left alone, as it was non-painful. However, they all knew it would eventually cause trouble and then some hard decision-making would be warranted.

I stared at the picture on the screen; unquestionably, it looked bad. I could see exactly where all the other vets were coming from. But then I could also see this man in front of me, increasingly desperate to do whatever it took to give his boxer another lease of life, asking help from anyone until he received the answer he wanted to hear. The lump was beginning to break on the surface and starting to smell. No more procrastination. 'I'll give it a go,' I said.

It is true that I like a surgical challenge, but you need to know your own, and nature's, limitations. I thought there was a chance here and so, after warning Murdo of the risks and possible complications, I booked a surgical slot for him the following week.

The big day came. A receptionist told me that, as Murdo was leaving the waiting room after dropping Milly for surgery, this hard-as-nails, caber-tossing macho man looked to be on the brink of tears.

In the end, the operation didn't require the removal of the leg, but it was impossible to close the defect by stretching and stitching the surrounding skin over the area where the lump had been. Significant aftercare was required. Initially the foot swelled up due to unavoidable damage to the circulation in the area. Thankfully, nature surmounted this obstacle herself; after a week or so, alternative circulation had established and the foot returned to normal.

About a week after that, the area was ready for phase two. Another operation was required: a skin graft, where I took pinches of skin from another area of the dog's body to graft over the defect and hurry healing along. Following that there was much toing and froing for bandage changes, and Murdo and Milly were regular visitors for a number of weeks. At each appointment, her hulk of an owner (who could no doubt hold a raging bull in a headlock) dealt so affectionately with his darling dog as he held her still for redressing of the wound.

Milly had soon become, shall we say, begrudgingly tolerant of veterinary attention. Of course, we have many reluctant patients; several step on the brakes at the door, or in the waiting room, and it can be easier just to lift and carry small dogs. The comical image left in my mind from the whole saga is of how Murdo dealt with the problem of Milly's unwillingness to enter the surgery. He would simply scoop up this 30kg dog with one of his enormous arms, tuck her under his armpit and saunter in and out of the practice as other clients might do with a tiny Chihuahua.

If you met a man of Murdo's frame and stature, you wouldn't be inclined to argue with him, and I'm so glad that I didn't argue back on the day he asked me to operate. Milly healed and recovered well, making a big man, with a big heart for his dog, very happy.

Chapter Sixteen

Leg and Bone Man

Every vet in our surgery is comfortable working across a range of animals presenting a wide host of issues, but we have each also developed 'our thing', a niche aspect of the job that we will invariably find ourselves tasked with whenever that particular type of work arises.

I'm the 'leg and bone' man, Tom is the equine vet, Ken and William tackle the cows' feet in the cow crate, Rebecca used to gravitate towards the birds, and Bridget (fairly unglamorously but nonetheless essentially) has a leaning towards dogs' bottoms.

Having our own areas of specialist interest is a really important part of what it takes to effectively run a remote mixed practice. We can be faced with almost any health problem, across a vast array of animal species, and we need to do our level best to provide a local service that can at least treat and fix most conditions. If we referred everything outside of the routine cases to a specialist down south, work could not only get quite dull for us, but frustrating for clients, who'd have to take days off work to travel significant distances. However, we don't have the time and resources for every single one of us to train up in everything, so the best solution we've found is for us each to acquire our own unique skillsets, and then bring them all to the table, as a team.

When they say I'm the leg and bone man, what they really mean is that, although I perform a wide variety of treatments and surgeries, I'm frequently the person undertaking the operations to fix skeletal problems – whether that be repairing nasty fractures or sorting out joint problems such as dislocations and cruciate disease. But just as Willie and Ken are more than bovine podiatrists (they are highly skilled farm vets), we all like to think of ourselves as good all-rounders, capable of tackling the array of routine cases that come our way, whatever the species.

The *Highland Vet* series has seen me conduct a few operations on dogs and their bones. A memorable case cropped up in the second season, and just recently, I was back working on that very same animal.

It was a couple of years ago when crofter Kirsteen was featured with her 11-month Border collie, Bob. He had a serious case of hip dysplasia. The hip is a ball-and-socket joint; the ball at the top of the thigh bone normally fits snuggly into a cup in the pelvis. In actuality, an X-ray showed that Bob's hips were so badly formed that, on each leg, the ball was barely covered by the cup at all. The left was the worst – the ball floating around the hip socket, grinding up against the lip of the cup, and causing him real pain.

Perhaps surprisingly, in both cats and dogs presenting with this condition, often the best course of action can be to cut off this ball of bone altogether, especially in lighter animals. The reason for this is twofold: firstly, it is an effective way of tackling the problem as it removes the source of the pain. With no bone grating on bone, tough but flexible scar tissue forms what I call a 'rubber joint'. This allows most animals to run around practically normally. The second reason is that the obvious alternative – referral for total hip-replacement surgery – is often prohibitively expensive for many pet owners, especially when considered against the efficacy of the more straightforward 'salvage' procedure, where the ball is simply removed.

The operation on Bob itself went well, with the removal of a very badly deformed left femoral head (the ball on the thigh bone) that resembled a lumpy little mushroom; but we always knew from the X-rays that we were going to have to operate on the other hip at some point in the future too. After all, the right hip was suffering the same problem, but wasn't yet giving Bob as much discomfort.

We planned on completing the second surgery just a couple of months later. Ordinarily, within reason, we encourage the dog to use the leg we've operated on, aiding the healing of a mobile 'rubber joint'. Typically, they will go back to bearing weight on it quickly, and then be walking almost normally after just two to three months. Cats, with their much lower weight, can achieve this within little over a month.

However, Bob really struggled to get into the rhythm of using the leg post-operatively. He was on pain relief, and I had regular chats with Kirsteen over the subsequent months, offering advice on home physiotherapy. But Bob often carried his leg, and it started to waste away. I wondered if he'd ever use it again and scratched my head at what on earth could be going on; the operation seemed to have gone as well as any other.

Many months later, Kirsteen was on the phone to another vet about a different matter, but she also asked to speak to me.

My relief was palpable: Bob was walking normally on the leg! Only now, nearly two years down the line from filming, have I been able to get on with removing his other femoral head on account of him now, quite evidently, struggling with pain on that side too.

Hopefully, Bob won't take anywhere near as long this time to get his leg going again. At any rate, I'll soon be calling his owner to keep track of his progress.

If I cast my mind back to myself as a boy, alongside my interest in animals, there was also a real fascination with how things worked and were put together. I'm sure this helped fuel my adult interest in surgery.

Back in the days when 'mechanical' reigned over 'electronic', inspired by my dad's partiality for the same thing, I would have no fear – indeed, I would positively enjoy – taking apart a gadget that had stopped working with the aim of fixing it. In that way I would learn how all the various bits inside fitted together, and how the machine worked, and then I would try to reassemble it again as if my whole dissection had never taken place.

At least once, I recall completing the task, only to discover that a component of the machine was still lying on the table in front of me, and yet, remarkably, the gadget still functioned perfectly well without it. It was a very early lesson that was equally applicable to surgery with animals. You can take out a spleen, you can remove a leg, the ball of a hip, or an eye, and an animal can find a way to carry on. In fact, more often than not, they will find ways to compensate for a missing body part; or even if function is less than it was, the animal's life is far better for the lack of a painful or diseased component.

Once I had made the decision to go into veterinary medicine, I found myself gravitating towards surgery. The 'carpentry with blood' aspect of orthopaedic work was particularly appealing. I never went down the route of full specialisation – I enjoy general practice – but about 12 years ago, I made the decision to take the leap into one of the big procedures we would often refer out to specialists.

The old adage 'There's a first time for everything' might be more applicable at the start of a career, to help people find the confidence to give things a go, with care and guidance, and not feel so fearful that they never learn by doing; but the issue with cutting through bones is that it is quite tricky to find those entry-level, gradual steps before taking on something pretty serious on a live animal. It might not really matter if you put the wrong milk in someone's coffee order, or give someone the wrong change, in the first week of a new job; but slicing through the wrong part of a body may not have reversable consequences for the animal, or your confidence (not to mention reputation) as a surgeon.

The big procedure I learnt was a type of 'tibial osteotomy' for treating cranial cruciate rupture. I can clearly remember my maiden osteotomy – the first time I ever cut through an animal's bone. I had been motivated to take up the training because I felt that by that point in my career, I had enough experience of surgery and general orthopaedics to make the leap. But, as much as I felt the need to keep pushing myself professionally, there was another obvious factor in my decision: we were having to refer all animals requiring an osteotomy to specialists. Specialists exist for good reason, and you must know when to defer to their greater experience and knowledge in the field they have chosen; but given that cruciate damage cropped up very frequently in the dogs local to us, the time seemed right for me to step up to the mark and offer this service in the far north.

I undertook a short training course in Sheffield, where I practised the procedure on plastic bones and learnt all the theory and practical pointers. On my return to Thurso, it wasn't long before we had a call from someone asking if I could offer such a procedure. They were soon to move to the area and their vet had suspected cruciate damage, though not confirmed it. I explained that I had just taken the course, but that I was yet to undertake an operation on a live animal. I was amazed that, despite having never met me, they had no reluctance to place their faith in me. A few weeks later, we admitted the dog into the surgery.

I can still see that dog in my mind's-eye hopping down the corridor towards me. *That's very lame,* I thought to myself. So lame, in fact, that it was almost incapable of bearing any weight on its injured leg. I might not have performed my fancy new surgery yet, but I had diagnosed enough cruciate ruptures to know something wasn't quite right here. *Surely that's more than just a cruciate rupture?* I pondered. *And if it is,* I added to my thought stream, *it's definitely not a good one to be starting with.*

My suspicions were proved correct on viewing the X-rays we then took. This dog had not ruptured its cruciate. It was hobbling because it had a nasty inoperable bone tumour. This poor animal was afflicted with a condition it could never hope to recover from. I called the owner and relayed the distressing news: their dog had to be put down.

They were obviously and understandably very upset, but what the owners said next was absolutely remarkable given what I had just told them. As they digested the awful news and composed their thoughts, they remembered that I had informed them I had not yet performed this operation other than on plastic bones. They asked me if I would like to keep their much-loved pet's body in order to practise the cruciate surgery on real flesh and bone. From their point of view, through tragic circumstances, it would be of some consolation that their dog would be benefitting fellow canines by helping me advance my surgical skills. I was extremely grateful.

The immense value of the donation of animals for the purposes of learning – and, likewise, of the generous folk who give up their bodies on death for medical students to further their training – can never be underestimated. From that point, I was later able to conduct my first tibial osteotomies on live dogs, and now I do very many each year.

Not wishing to pigeonhole myself, I do all sorts of varied surgical procedures, boney and otherwise, and I enjoy the wider breadth of indoor and outdoor work that a mixed practice provides; but with respect to orthopaedics, as the years passed, the jobs I could manage broadened, and it wasn't too long before I was the de-facto local leg and bone man. There are still the really tricky cases that I inevitably have to refer, but I'm really glad I've been able to add to the spectrum of what we can offer in Thurso.

Being a vet does have an obvious practical side to it. Yes, you need to be academic and scientifically minded to be capable enough to study and retain knowledge and then use it to make sound judgements regarding diagnosis and treatment, but you also need to be prepared for the very hands-on nature of the job.

For me, it is that combination of an intellectual puzzle *and* a challenge of fine motor skills that really fires me up about being a vet. Performing surgery, particularly orthopaedic surgery, is where I find an optimal combination of those aspects. Fixing anything is very satisfying, but when it is a living creature, the satisfaction is immense. I'm certain human doctors and surgeons must feel the same.

There is no obvious one thing that makes a good leg and bone surgeon, but a good dollop of bravery goes a long way, because ultimately you know that you, the animal and their owner will all have to live with the consequences of the decision and the action you took when you reached that point of no return. Oddly, as my career progresses and confidence, experience and wisdom build, it's often the managing of anxiety surrounding my own expectations of myself that remains one of the biggest challenges to surmount.

It is a sad fact that, no matter what your level of skill, there will always be those rare times when an operation doesn't have an optimal outcome. What's hard, though, is accepting that simple statistical fact for what it is and remembering there are often multiple factors that feed into such scenarios. You must try to unburden yourself of the apprehension about something that is inevitable if you're going to take on complex procedures.

I console myself that worrying, even about things you can't control, is probably a good sign of a caring vet; but it doesn't help you sleep well some nights.

Chapter Seventeen

When It's Raining Cats and Dogs

The coronavirus pandemic, with its 'stay at home' lockdowns, has seen the past couple of years manifest the steepest rise in British pet ownership during my time in practice, and the prices of cats and dogs have shot up too. We are a nation of cat and dog lovers, so it should be no surprise that those species dominate the domestic pet market. It is estimated there are a staggering 24 million cats and dogs in people's homes today. In Europe, only Germany has more dogs than us.

As a vet practice that sees pets, that obviously means we are seeing more of them than ever, and the more dramatic cases punctuate days that are otherwise filled with less demanding issues: vaccinations, routine checks and standard procedures.

Following are a few day-to-day tasks and common presentations relating to our canine and feline companions that, I'm sure, if you are an owner, you may well be familiar with:

Dog and cat neutering: We perform castration (the removal of a male cat or dog's testicles) and spaying (the removal of a female's uterus and ovaries) many times a year. The most obvious benefit of these operations is that they will stop your animal from producing unwanted offspring. It is worth noting there are other pros and cons to such procedures, which are best weighed on an individual animal basis.

Pregnancy: Owners of bitches in pup often like pregnancy confirmed by an ultrasound scan and are reassured to see that all is well. But left long enough, pregnancy confirms itself with obvious outward signs – abdominal enlargement and mammary gland development. However, I have experienced two extreme scenarios in this vein. Let me explain. Scenario one: the owner is certain their bitch is pregnant due to her increase in girth, but unfortunately, I have to disappoint them when I scan the belly. Wishful thinking on their part had led them to feed their dog more in the hope she had little pups inside demanding her resources, but in the end, she was just a bit chubbier. Scenario two: a client brings in a dog, either worried that she has a serious illness or asking for dietary advice due to unexplained weight gain. The expression on their face is priceless when I break the news that their dog's condition is perfectly natural and that in a few weeks' time they'll find themselves with several extra little pets!

Lumpectomies: A lumpectomy is the surgical removal of a lump. For obvious reasons, owners become concerned about the appearance of lumps and bumps. They can range from benign fatty growths that can be left alone, right through to scary cancerous types, and it is seldom apparent on outward appearance where on that spectrum a lump may lie. Even some benign lumps can cause annoyance that justifies surgery. A wart is hardly more than a cosmetic issue in many cases, but on an eyelid, for example, it can rub and cause discomfort. For this we pull out a brilliantly simple piece of protective kit in the form of a household teaspoon: carefully slid underneath the eyelid to protect the dog's eyeball as we work the wart away with a scalpel.

Eye ulcers: These occur commonly too. Sophie, a cat filmed for the TV, needed treatment for this condition. We will treat ulcers rather counterintuitively; we damage the ulcerated area further by scraping it with a needle, which stimulates a bodily healing response. Then we cover the eye by stitching over the animal's own third eyelid (a 'nictitating membrane' found in some fish, amphibians, reptiles, birds and mammals but not in humans), which acts as a fantastic natural bandage over the eye.

Stitch-up jobs: When dogs, and occasionally cats, have cut themselves on anything from branches to fences, and broken glass to sharp pieces of metal in the river.

Skin and ear disease: Itchy dogs and gungy ears – oh, how our days would be incomplete without them!

Sickness and diarrhoea: Once again, never a day goes by …

Dental issues: Domestic pets don't brush their teeth like humans do. Chewing activity can help keep them clean, but, unless you brush them as faithfully as brushing your own (special pet toothpaste and brushes are available) then sooner or later, dental work will be required. Routine descaling, along with extraction of diseased and damaged teeth, is regular work for a pet vet.

Anal glands: What we simply call anal glands are more correctly called anal sacs. They are pouches of glandular tissue that sit either side of the anus of cats and dogs and form part of the natural scenting found so commonly in the animal kingdom. Dogs love the smell of each other's bottoms, but the liquid from these pungent pouches is utterly repulsive to the human nose. Frequently the sacs overfill or are unable to empty, and this is where a vet with gloved fingers comes to the fore (or should I say, to the rear?).

The obvious signs of blocked anal sacs can include: a woeful whiff from the animal's hind end; constant bum licking (and hence bad breath); or 'scooting', whereby the animal will bum-shuffle along your carpet, leaving a horrific stinky smear. The procedure to milk the anal sacs to void them of their grotty goo is fairly straight-forward. Some can be relieved by pressure from the outside, but if not, then you slip your finger into the anus, locate the grape-like sacs, usually just on the inside, and give them a firm but gentle squeeze. Their rancid contents smell like rotting fish and can be smooth in texture through to granular or almost oatmeal-like. They can be quite explosive as well, and so you cup your hand over the anus to avoid the malodorous mixture from spraying all over you. Inattention at this point is ill-advised. I have squirted the stuff onto my clothing and up the wall on numerous occasions. I even hit my face recently (saved by the Covid regulations, my mask took the brunt of it). But, as is so often the case in life, there are always people considerably worse off than yourself: one of our vets, who shall remain nameless,* ran to the toilet and vomited after he was once sprayed squarely in his open mouth.

---

* It was Ken.

There are certain occupational hazards inherent in examining dogs and cats that you just have to accept as part of the job. Often, they will urinate or defecate all over you due to the stress of an examination. Close encounters with pee and poo are something you just learn to get used to.

I remember once, one of the nurses had successfully managed to restrain a small dog for an examination, and when everything was finally in order, she innocently reached inside the front of her tunic and discovered the gift of a freshly formed faecal frankfurter deposited in the pocket.

I, too, have fallen foul of faeces when out on numerous farms. Ordinarily, a farmer will shout something useful like 'Watch yersel'!' or 'Timber!' to warn the unsuspecting vet working on a cow's hind feet that they are about to receive a very unwelcome head adornment. At one place, however, the farmer was negligent of the usual courtesies and seemed to find it funny to just let his cow cock its tail and land me a pat on the head. The cow muck then slowly dribbled down my neck and under my collar. That story has long since been immortalised in the memories of hundreds of local children, thanks to my primary schoolteacher wife, whose six-year-olds find it, frankly, hilarious.

Calving cows brings further opportunity to receive Scotland's worst spray tan. You are right in the firing line when conducting a vaginal birth, and, given that calving puts huge pressure on the cow's rectum as the calf squeezes past on its way out, it can easily relieve its compressed contents all over the vet in charge. I've been hit full in the face on multiple occasions, so the taste of cow dung is not unfamiliar to me. While I'm on the subject, conducting cow caesareans is another grand opportunity for a good coating of bodily fluids. A cow that probably hasn't coughed in weeks seems to choose the moment you're peering into its open flank to release a hearty cough from the depths of its being. The volcanic expulsion of the fluid and blood that has accumulated in its abdomen during the operation leaves you peppered with hideous blotches, as if afflicted by a highly contagious tropical disease.

The other obvious way a cat or a dog might display its displeasure in the surgery is through aggression. Of course, it varies from animal to animal, but you usually get some forewarning that they might be about to tell you off with their claws or teeth. As a vet, you learn to read the cues, giving yourself a chance to back off, give them some space, and then reassess your approach. Even so, when you've been a vet for long enough, you will have been bitten by a cat or dog on at least one occasion.

In the same way that cats themselves present with abscesses when they have been bitten by other cats, they can do the same to a human, on account of the infective bacteria in their mouths. I've had at least a couple of unpleasant bites in my time: one was treated with antibiotics; another I let boil into an abscess before squeezing out the pus in the shower. Neither left any lasting aftermath.

Dog bites, though, they can really do you some damage. A cuddly and loving pet in relation to its familiar owner may react badly to having a stranger in its personal space, especially one who stuck a needle in it last time they met. Understandably, they feel threatened and display a need for self-preservation, so be on your guard.

One particularly memorable dog bite happened when a very on-edge and stressed collie came to see me. 'Fight or flight' was very much tuned to 'fight' for this dog. It reacted with snarling and snapping as I approached, so I backed off, ceding the space, as was only sensible. This is normally the dog's cue to back down, but it didn't play by the book; it lunged forward, and before it was checked by the owner holding the leash, it sunk its teeth into the hand I instinctively raised to protect myself. It was a nasty bite, certainly the worst I've had from any dog, and took some time to heal.

Although dogs undoubtedly have different personalities, many cases of bad behaviour have a simple root: human neglect or well-intentioned ignorance. Adequate and sensible socialisation as a puppy is critical for a dog to learn about the world and how to interact with it. Often, inappropriate behaviour stems from poor socialisation during those important early weeks. Additionally, many bad behaviours in dogs are reinforced, or even taught, unwittingly by the humans they interact with. When problems arise, animal behaviour therapy is often sought to retrain a dog's way of thinking and responding in certain contexts. In reality, it can be just as crucial to retrain the human to respond to the dog appropriately in certain contexts.

Chapter Eighteen

A Hole in the Head

If a dog picks a fight with a vet, you might not wish to place bets on who would come off the worst; but when a dog comes up against a heavy moving vehicle, the odds are most definitely stacked against it. Earlier this year, a rather dramatic case made this point all too clearly.

Up until about midday, it had been a fairly typical day. After completing a big bone operation in the morning, I had moved on to all the miscellaneous tasks and paperwork that are always waiting in the wings, when Alison, our receptionist, relayed the substance of an urgent call. I am always more than happy to skip any pending admin to step up to something more stimulating. Vet David had just entered the office too, and, on overhearing the conversation, he hovered at the top of the wee flight of stairs that head down to the kitchen.

A dog had been hit by a bus on the edge of town, but we knew little more than the approximate location. It sounded serious, potentially disastrous. David and I looked at each other. 'I'll come with you,' he said. We both knew from experience that two pairs of hands are far better than one in such circumstances. The dog could be writhing in pain or behaving erratically – not easy to treat at the scene without help, nor to function as an ambulance without someone to restrain the patient in the car.

We ran to grab various useful items like a stretcher and pain-relieving medication, then hopped into my car and made our way across town.

A collision with a bus! Would the dog still be alive? There was a real possibility that wasn't going to be the case. The journey to the scene was only a short one – nowhere in Thurso is too far from the surgery – yet halfway there, our progress was thwarted by a long chain of cars barely moving in front of us on the main road.

Ironic, I thought. *I bet that's due to the very accident we are trying to get to.* Unfortunately, vets don't get issued with blue flashing lights!

Both of us were itching to get to the injured dog. The car hadn't been stationary in the queue for long before David and I looked at each other again, the same thought going through our minds. 'I'll get out and run the rest of it,' he said. 'See you there in a few minutes.' David was half my age, so I was glad my decision to drive saved me from the sprint. He grabbed a stethoscope and tore off along the pavement in the direction of the accident.

As my car eventually approached the location, I found no major crash scene and the bus had already moved on. Just a small group of people were gathered around a black-and-white Border collie, lying motionless at a road junction. I turned in, stopped the car and jumped out.

David was ready to fill me in. He had administered pain relief and assessed the situation. The collie had been practically comatose since his arrival, but thankfully it was still alive. *Well, at least for now*, I thought.

I had a quick look at the only obvious wound. An irregular hole was visible in the top of the dog's head. On closer inspection, it was apparent that it was not simply skin-deep: the skull itself had caved in at that point. I peered into it and wondered whether I was gazing right into where the brain should be. It was hard to be certain of the anatomical points without an X-ray, but if the fragment of bone at the bottom of the chasm was squashing into his brain tissue, the likelihood of survival was very slim.

We carefully put the dog on a stretcher, and David sat with him in the car as we travelled back to the surgery. We now had a name for our charge, although he was in no state to respond to it. Sweep was a young working farm collie who had a second home in town. On the breeze, he'd sniffed a faint but irresistible whiff of a bitch on heat and had made a run for it. If his head was still capable of any thoughts, without doubt he'd now be wishing he'd controlled his urges. I reckon he'd rather have taken on the hard head of the most cantankerous tup on his farm than the front end of a bus!

Back at the surgery, David reassessed Sweep's vital signs and X-rayed the skull. He lay completely immobile for the X-rays. The pain relief given at the scene would have doped him to some degree, but our fear was that he was still out for the count due to the impact to his head. Other vital signs – pulse, respiration – were all good; the focus for now was on the neurological injury – the damage to his brain.

I was called in to assess the X-ray images and was relieved to find that the skull fracture had just missed the cranium – the brain case – and was into Sweep's frontal sinus. This sinus is a natural air-filled cavity within the skull, like those we humans have and which clog up during a cold. But any optimism had to remain very cautious; the trauma may not have fractured the bones around the brain, but the impact could nevertheless have caused a lot of collateral damage, possibly even brain-bleeding. Supportive treatment, pain relief and monitoring were all we could do for now. It was a waiting game. Would he regain consciousness or slip deeper and deeper away from us?

I was on call that night and so monitoring Sweep and our other inpatients was my job until morning. Other vets and nurses later admitted they did not expect to find him still with us on their arrival the next day. I assessed his consciousness as the evening wore on and, to my amazement and delight, by bedtime he was looking at me, aware I was present, and even enjoying a little belly tickle. His brain had evidently undergone a severe rattling, causing swelling that was apparently subsiding. A continued increase of pressure within his skull, due to any bleeding, now seemed very unlikely. We could finally relax a little.

The nurses were overjoyed not only to find Sweep sitting up and fully responsive the next day, but also to discover that he was a big softie and very easy to work with. Vet Fiona was on duty in theatre that morning and assessed Sweep as being in a fit enough state to undergo minor surgery for the hole in his head and also to have X-rays taken of his right foreleg, which, now he was conscious and mobile, was obviously causing him trouble too.

I was enjoying my day off, having been on call the previous night, and Jennifer and I were walking Milis and appreciating some Highland fresh air. Halfway up an incline leading to the stunning clifftop path at Dunnet, my phone pinged in my pocket. Being of a certain generation, I'm perfectly capable of ignoring text messages until I'm ready to deal with them, but I decided to take a look. There on my screen was an X-ray image of Sweep's leg, sent by Fiona. Not only had he fractured his skull, but the two bones in the lower portion of his front leg – the radius and ulna – had been snapped too. I typed back some advice, secretly glad of the breather it afforded me during my short ascent. After tidying up the head injury, Fiona would have to discuss options for treatment of the leg with the owner, ranging from amputation to stabilising the bones with a metal plate and screws.

On surgically exploring the wound on the top of Sweep's head, Fiona judged that little could be done about the broken skull bone, so the fragments were removed. The skin was stitched and would heal to leave a soft spot below; perhaps surprisingly, that would be of little concern. Fiona also removed small pieces of blue stuff from the wound, they obviously weren't original bits of Sweep's head; she concluded they must have been shards of paint from the bus. For me, such a finding triggers recollection of a time when, as a new graduate, I was called to a horse 'the morning after the night before'. The mare had escaped her field and been hit on the road. Remarkably, there were no broken bones, only flesh wounds. More remarkably, there had been no major human casualties, which unfortunately is not always the case when collisions with such large animals occur. As I probed the damaged tissue, I felt my metal forceps grate against a hard material and soon extracted several fragments of windscreen glass from her lacerations before stitching them up.

Sweep's owner wanted to take the option that would offer the quickest route to healing with the least chance of complications, so that he could return him to work as soon as possible. That meant surgery and metal implants. I didn't have a suitable bone plate for his leg and so, with the help of the X-ray images, I measured up and ordered one on next-day delivery.

It isn't always necessary to fix both the radius and ulna when the two of them fracture simultaneously, as so often happens. I planned to apply a metal plate to the radius only. It was a bit of a fiddle to bring its fragments together, and then to site the plate in the ideal position along the bone's surface in order to receive the screws. Somewhat counterintuitively, it is not always required or appropriate to fit broken bones back together with the perfection desired when supergluing pieces of a valuable vase. But this case was one where I had the satisfaction of seeing the irregular edges come together like placing the final gratifying piece of a jigsaw puzzle.

The plate was what is known in the trade as a 'dynamic compression plate'; in this type of plate the screw holes are cleverly shaped such that, when a screw is inserted, the fracture-site is marginally squeezed together, thus increasing stability and efficiency of healing. Almost as if I'd planned it, by drawing the radius into alignment, the ends of the broken ulna running alongside it were realigned too, and would, I hoped, heal without additional fixation; the now-rigid radius would naturally splint its companion during the healing period.

What a turnaround for the dog I'd first met unconscious by the roadside. Sweep's remarkable progress had been a real team effort. Within just a few days, if you'd asked Sweep, he would have told you he was ready to get back to working with sheep; it was fair to say, thanks to his natural exuberance, he was definitely a little too keen to use his leg. And incredibly, he had no lasting mental effects from a collision that, in all reason, had every possibility of proving fatal. He was eventually persuaded to take a two-month period of calm convalescence while his leg healed, but getting that concept through his skull – even though part of it wasn't as thick as it used to be – wasn't so easy; he was raring to go!

Chapter Nineteen

A Royal Visit

The grand old Castle of Mey sits on the north coast a little over 13 miles east of Thurso. The Queen Mother purchased it in a semi-derelict state back in 1952, not long after the death of her husband, King George VI. She had first seen the place for sale while spending time with her friends Commander and Lady Doris Vyner, who lived just along the coast at Dunnet, and it was widely known that she loved Caithness.

Having secured the castle, the Queen Mother would continue to have an annual summer holiday there for the next five decades, with her last visit taking place when she had reached a remarkable 101 years of age; but, before she died in 2002, she gifted the castle to a charitable trust. Overseen by her grandson Prince Charles, the trust opened the castle's buildings and grounds to the public, and maintained a herd of Aberdeen Angus cattle and a flock of North Country Cheviot sheep with the aims of preservation, education and public engagement in the local community.

Once I knew that Prince Charles – or the Duke of Rothesay, to give him his Scottish title – was planning to pay our surgery a visit, I was asked to keep it all hush-hush until close to the date. However, when staff knew a VIP would be visiting, it didn't take the investigative nous of Hercule Poirot to work out who it was likely to be. Firstly, Prince Charles is a regular to the county; he was very fond of his grandmother and was keen to preserve her legacy at the castle first-hand. Secondly, the trust closes the Castle of Mey for the same period each summer, when it becomes, once more, a royal residence.

The secrecy, quite sensibly, was all about preventing crowds in view of Covid, but if the cat had really been let out of the bag prematurely, I doubt there would have been anything to worry about. There's a healthy level-headedness to folk up here. Although there may be as much interest in and respect for the royals as elsewhere, people are unlikely to whip themselves up into a fever over a visit from one of them. Perhaps that was among the reasons why the Queen Mother enjoyed Caithness as much as she did: she was permitted to do what she pleased, when she pleased, without the intensity of the media scrutiny and fanfare the royal family tend to generate with their every movement in the more southerly parts of our fair kingdom. She was even known to drive herself into town for a stroll around. Over 20 years ago now, my wife and daughter came across the Queen Mother outside Woolworths one day.

It was only a couple of years after the Queen Mother had passed away that I had my first contact with Prince Charles. Involvement in the local community was a factor in this royal appointment, but for reasons other than my role as a vet.

Outside of my often-preoccupying veterinary work, I like to play, arrange and compose music. I find, like surgery, playing music utilises that optimal fusion of brain and body. It is a family affair: Jennifer plays the violin and harp, and our two daughters were encouraged in musical pursuits from a young age and have excelled on their chosen instruments of violin and piano. My regular venue is our local church, where songs ancient and modern are sung in praise, with me, usually, on the piano (unless our youngest is home, in which case I give way to her superior skill and bop along on the guitar or bass).

As a family we have enjoyed making music together in many styles over the years, including Scottish traditional music, where the accompaniment would often receive a souped-up 'Guy treatment', which at least one of us enjoyed. In a small community, it didn't take long before we were 'on the circuit', performing at local evening events and charity functions. When the girls were young the appeal of a family playing together seemed to get the wholesome 'aah' factor. Then, as the girls became more proficient, they moved to the fore as Mum and Dad stepped back a little. (And comments like 'Mum, you're singing a little flat' became more frequent.)

I recall one year in early June when the girls were in their mid-teens, I was on call the night before they were due to perform in Wick at the annual Caithness Music Festival. This seemed ideal as my night shift meant that I had the following day off. However, old Murphy and his law once again paid me a visit. I was called to a calving not long before my 8.30am clock-off time and, in accordance with the rules, it was my job to start and finish as the call had come in on my time. I had to be in Wick sitting at a piano to accompany my daughter by 10am. Murphy then dealt me another blow: the cow needed a Caesar, of course.

I couldn't believe it. Of all the days! I knew I wouldn't make it, so I phoned the surgery just as they were opening for the morning and asked them to send a vet to relieve me. Fortunately, there was someone available to shoot out to my rescue. In the meantime, the cow was my responsibility, so I started the operation, got the calf out, and started stitching. *Hurry up, hurry up!* I thought, trying to keep a professional exterior as I internally willed my colleague to arrive.

Once backup appeared, as if competing in some surgical relay race, I passed the baton – or rather the needle – to my fellow vet and I sped off to Wick. On arrival I dashed into the toilets to freshen up and inspect myself in the mirror (always sensible after a farm call to check for those unsightly blood splats). I was in the nick of time. With barely a moment to think, I was at the piano, vamping merrily away as my daughter expertly bowed her violin for the audience and adjudicator.

Normally I suffer a fair dose of performance anxiety, and I feel it worse when accompanying at an important occasion; the pressure to play well for the soloist's sake is immense. (I once lost my place playing the piano along to a Vivaldi violin duet. I never found my place again, and even as I write, reliving those scarring few minutes is getting me in a flap!)

What was interesting about this morning was how I had no nerves at all; I had never played so well and with such cool. Occupying my mind with simply getting to the venue on time, along with not having to wait around with my daughter, getting nervous together as other competitors played, was the best remedy for performance nerves. However, Jennifer was a wreck after having sat there waiting and waiting, not knowing whether I'd make it at all!

Returning to my first engagement with Prince Charles: it came about by way of a combination of my faith and my musical interests. One afternoon during my early years in Thurso, I answered the telephone, and Jennifer could gather from what was being said that she and I were being asked to play and sing at an event, a church service. Nothing new there. She heard the date and urgently whispered, 'You can't do that date, Guy, you're on call', to which I scribbled 'PRINCE CHARLES' in large letters on the paper in front of me. Through the powers of non-verbal, wide-eyed communication, it was immediately agreed that we would surely find another vet willing to cover my duties for the couple of hours required for us to perform!

Canisbay Parish Church is a lovely old building overlooking the Pentland Firth. There, guitar in hand, my usual anxiety was eased somewhat as the heir to the throne smiled encouragingly. A quartet comprising myself, my wife, and a couple of friends sang for the royals. We held our nerves together enough to perform well on that day. I even slipped in one of my own original compositions based on Psalm 51.

I didn't get an opportunity to ask Prince Charles if he had enjoyed what he'd heard – his suited entourage were rather keen on ushering him out of the church as soon as the service was over – but Camilla did have a moment to come over and thank us, even revealing that she'd dabbled with the guitar herself, in the days before her duty to the Crown had changed her life's path.

During Prince Charles's annual stays in the county, he does like to busy himself with various appearances in the community, as well as visits to places he finds of particular interest. Each year, Lord Thurso, the Lord Lieutenant of Caithness – the Queen's personal representative in our area – supplies the Prince with a list of potential options of engagements with which to fill his time. I can imagine Prince Charles, fountain pen in hand, putting a little tick next to the things he would like to do. Well, this summer, he ticked 'Visit Thurso veterinary surgery'.

I didn't know any of that initially; I just got a slightly cryptic message from the surgery saying that Lord Thurso himself wished to speak with me – to which my natural response was 'Oh dear', and a swift rack of the brains to consider whether I'd done anything worthy of banishment to the Tower. In the event, however, our chat went really well. Lord Thurso, though unsurprisingly a very well-spoken and highly educated man, is friendly and pleasantly down to earth. He came to the surgery offering advice, and listening to my ideas, as to what the Prince might like to see and chat about as we mocked up a royal tour around our premises.

Thanks to Covid, we were limited with our indoor options so we tried to design as much of the tour as possible to take place out in the car park and in the lambing shed. We set up the hydraulic cow foot-crate, with vet William demonstrating, and had a few small groups of people scattered around our outdoor spaces for the Prince to interact with.

I had a little jangle of nerves on the morning of the visit, just about silly things like *What if the Prince trips over something?* or *What if William tells one of his inappropriate jokes?* or *What if an asteroid randomly hits the practice?* But it really couldn't have gone much better. It was the middle of summer, but that doesn't preclude dreich days entirely in Scotland; there was a light drizzle in the air. Still, the Prince didn't seem to notice it. Spirits were high as he swept in with his entourage. Of course, there were security officials and police, but they were all so courteous and in the background.

Prince Charles was wearing a red tartan kilt and green woollen socks and was clearly in a very genial mood. He was in no desperate hurry to leave and took his time with the tour, speaking to everyone. He donned a face mask to comply with regulations so he could have a look within the surgery buildings too. It certainly didn't feel like he was paying lip service to his duties at all; he was genuinely interested in our work and revealed himself to be very knowledgeable about farming, cattle and their care.

Face to face with number one in line to the throne, you'd think we might have been all wide-eyed and bumbling our words, but in spite of the secrecy and therefore heightened anticipation in the build-up to his visit, Prince Charles himself put all of us very much at ease. Personally, I was eager that the tour ran without a glitch, and I guess that tension has left me a little vague on what we actually spoke about. I didn't embarrass him by asking if he remembered me singing all those years ago; he will have seen millions of faces in the interim. I asked whether he and Camilla had dogs; he chatted to each staff member in turn about their own role within the practice; and he even spoke to Jennifer about her work at the school. Jennifer had been grafted in to take photos on behalf of the practice and wound up as the sole remaining photographer after the press pack had moved on to be ready and waiting at the Prince's next location. Appropriately, that subsequent engagement was a visit to the recently renovated former residence of his grandmother's friends, the Vyners, atop Dunnet Head.

No doubt the Duke of Rothesay is very well practised in small talk with the public, but there was never a moment when the discussion felt stilted, forced or awkward. A big surprise of the day was, really, just how easy the conversation felt at times, without ever detracting from the fact that his visit was also a huge honour for our small-town veterinary practice up here in the north.

Autumn

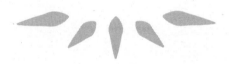

Chapter Twenty

This Wild Life

Even in a place like Caithness, where it can feel like wildlife is all around us – secretly staring from within the trees or gazing up from a riverbed; looking across from the sea or peering loftily from a cliff face – genuine close encounters with wild animals are still very rare.

Of course, a notable quality of any wild animal is its ability to use its stealth, speed, camouflage or heightened awareness to stay out of our reach. If you put in the time to sit in a hide and wait at dawn or dusk, your patience may be rewarded as a rare sight unfolds in your presence; but more often than not, an encounter will be unexpected and fleeting: a fresh print in the mud or a sudden flash of fur or feather in the headlights. To actually hold a wild creature in your hand is truly exceptional. It always leaves an impression, especially on the very young.

My first physical contact with a wild animal came at the age of nine or ten. Our family heard a scuffle in the garden and we found our cat toying, in a fiendishly feline way, with what turned out to be a young weasel. We managed to intervene before a fatal level of torment had occurred, and my two brothers and I took it upon ourselves to rehabilitate this poor wee victim.

We had no idea of its gender, but let's say 'he' didn't seem to have suffered any significant physical harm; he just appeared stressed, disorientated and presumably a little sore. In our garage, a box was turned on its side and, with a mesh grill fitted over the opening and newspaper laid inside, it became a hospital cage.

We fed him bits of meat my mum provided from the kitchen; our family had enough general knowledge between us to know that a weasel is a carnivore. You must remember, in the seventies you couldn't ask Google, 'What does a weasel eat?' (For your interest, I have just done that, and the answer is mice, voles, rabbits and frogs, among other small prey.)

I felt such a thrill and sense of awe when handling the little creature. A real wild animal in my own hands! I presume my parents had told us to wear gardening gloves, I don't know that I would have had the sense at that age. I recall wondering why he wasn't immediately grateful and happy to be the friend of the hand that fed him. At each approach, he initially bit defensively at the gloves before settling down. It was an important lesson to learn as a child: this was a wild animal and domestication in 24 hours just wasn't going to happen!

To be honest, it hadn't really occurred to me that I was playing vet, but in hindsight, to have such an animal in my care was likely to have been a hitherto unrecognised step on the path that led to what I do today. A year or so after that, in my final year at primary school, I had another opportunity to play vet. This time, I was onstage. My friend Craig and I enacted a silly sketch we had written for all the parents and pupils where, along with other capers, we treated a cat (for this we used a pyjama case) that had been flattened on the road by reinflating it with a bicycle pump.

My sense of humour has not improved, unfortunately, since those days, but thankfully my feline-resuscitation skills have.

Within only a couple of days, when it was apparent all was well with our wriggly companion, we decided to set him free. Although reluctant to lose our new little friend and the interest he had brought to our lives, we instinctively knew that a longer period of captivity would have been wrong: let wild animals roam wild. In the meantime, using the limited resources of my animal reference books (most of which I still have today), I had created my own little home project on weasels. I loved to draw, so I suspect more of the pages were taken up by pictures than words, and the latter would certainly have benefitted from a run through spell-check, had it existed.

My little brother tells me he can still recall feeling very upset at having to say goodbye. Our house backed onto a golf course and nearby farmland, so together we carried the weasel in its box a short distance to the corner of a field by a small brook, having taken a guess that his family may have originated in that vicinity. On smelling the fresh air, he ran swiftly and cheerfully through the grass for a couple of metres, and then (it is possible my memory romanticises the following few moments) he stopped, turned his head and looked back at us over his left shoulder.

I feel he would have saluted if he could, as if to say, 'Cheerio, chaps, and thanks.' Then he scurried off into the deeper grass and that was the last we saw of him. I do wonder if he made it, found a mate and had a family; I like to think that there exists today a large extended clan of direct descendants of the small furry friend that made such an impression on me at the time.

In relation to our domestic workload at the surgery, a wild animal is a rarity. When it comes to the question of what can be done for a wild creature, we have to be realistic about the chances of a successful outcome. My weasel encounter as a child was exceptional, not simply because of its utter singularity but also because it ended so positively, with the animal making a full recovery and heading back with vigour into its natural habitat. Sadly, in most cases, the very fact we are able to get close enough to even handle a wild creature means it is almost certainly well on its way out.

The hard reality of the natural world is that it is an uncompromising crucible, where the line between life and death is often very fine. Autumn in the Highlands is the last chance for many species to feast; the days become shorter, and soon the long winter nights will see that the opportunities to find and forage for food recede quite dramatically.

Small mammals and birds turn to berry-filled hedgerows, and huge flocks of wild greylag geese arrive from Iceland – alongside wigeons, barnacle geese and many other migratory wildfowl species – to find food and shelter on our lochs and intertidal flats. Autumn is also the time for one of Scotland's most spectacular wildlife events of the year: the red deer rut, when the amply antlered stags engage in violent battles with their mating rivals and roar out defensive warning calls at dawn and dusk.

Predatory species can do serious damage to their prey all year round, and so can humans, who cause a multitude of injuries to wildlife with their cars, litter and pollution. Even just the way we build our homes can present problems; we concrete and tarmac over formerly wild habitats, and I'm sure we've all heard the thud of a bird as it unwittingly flies into one of our glass windowpanes.

Autumn can bring stunning days to the Highlands, with golden colours in turning leaves, but there may also be sudden cold snaps, storms and very fierce winds. Animals are instinctively more aware of seasonal changes than us, but they are also much more vulnerable to those abrupt changes in weather, and that climatological savagery can see many animal species, especially birds, come a cropper.

The question we must always try to answer as vets, before we even consider whether to treat a wild animal, is: will it survive reintroduction to the wild? If, after our assessment of its condition, the answer is no, then really, we have to think about what would be gained from treating and releasing it. Better a swift and pain-less euthanasia than a drawn-out death of starvation, or a stressful demise in the claws or teeth of a predator it stands no chance of escaping. In some circumstances there may be the possibility of protection in a sanctuary, but (and sorry to depress you) by far the majority of wildlife cases end with us deciding that the most logical and ethical thing to do is put the poor creature down. However, that's not to say that we never have any real success stories.

In the event of finding a wild animal in distress, in Scotland the first port of call should be the SSPCA, but frequently, members of the public just call the vets. We will then liaise with the charity regarding treatment and rehabilitation. On other occasions the SSPCA inspector will have been contacted by the public and will bring the animal directly to us if it requires our expertise. The charity has facilities for prolonged rehabilitation, but we have occa-sionally released animals ourselves after a short stay in the surgery.

We've had all sorts come through our doors over the years, from a pipistrelle bat with a tear in its wing to sick hedgehogs found listless in people's gardens. This year, *The Highland Vet* even featured an exceptionally unusual story in the shape of a young red deer that had taken refuge within farmer Ray's outbuildings. The deer was found very unwell and had been sheltering in one of his barns. In this case, vet William suspected a serious viral infection, which he attempted to treat. The series has also twice featured baby otters: one that was sent on to the SSPCA, and another that sadly didn't make it. And then there are all the wild birds.

As you have already learnt earlier in this book, small birds have an especially high risk of anaesthetic-related death. With wild birds, even if they initially seem quite lively, the stress of captivity and handling can be enough to send them to their demise. The general advice from the specialised rehabilitation centre Raptor Rescue is to try to remember that not all birds you find on the ground are sick or injured. A young bird will often have a misadventure while learning to fly, and, if left well alone, its parents will return for it. Indeed, young owls are well known for their ability to actually climb trees to make it back to the roost.

If you feel the need to handle a bird, you are advised to catch it using a large towel and then place it in a cardboard box with the towel or a piece of carpet in it, just to give them something to grip on to. Close the lid securely (while making sure there is some ventilation for the bird to breathe, of course!); the darkness will help keep the bird calm and reduce the chances of it damaging itself further in a panicked attempt at flight. Then call a specialist independent rescue centre or the SSPCA (or its equivalent in your country). You need to be very careful handling any bird. Firstly, be aware that their faeces may contain bacteria that could infect you. Wear gloves or at least wash your hands well afterwards. Moreover, they can injure you: the talons of birds of prey can be fiercely strong, and larger fish-catching wild birds with long necks, such as the cormorant, present another danger. Their cobra-like motion and razor-sharp beaks have been known to maim well-meaning members of the public; a man in Wales was even blinded while rescuing a gannet. When we handle them, we ensure the neck is held behind the head and we've even taken to wearing safety goggles.

Birds are tricky customers at the best of times. Earlier this year, a series of gales brought vet Rebecca a job with a tawny owl, injured after having been blown down a chimney; and a barn owl was brought to the surgery for vet Eilidh to examine. I once went on a 'wild owl chase' off the back of a very vague phone call. I repeatedly drove and then walked up and down a stretch of road where an owl was reported to be struggling by the roadside. I eventually managed to locate the tawny owl on the overgrown verge, and on return to the surgery I successfully administered fluids to the bird via my first intraosseous drip (into the bone).

We've also treated swans and buzzards, and once we even had a puffin come through the doors. It wasn't sick or damaged and certainly wasn't as cute as it looked; it had a bit of a feisty side to it and, memorably, bit one of our nurses before its successful release across the bay from the nearby port of Scrabster. This year, for the first time, I had two kestrels in quick succession: one had a nasty mouth infection, which I tried to treat with antibiotics (but, unfortunately, it didn't pull through); the other was quite weak and lethargic but was eventually rehabilitated at a raptor rehabilitation centre in Sutherland and released back into the wild to fight another day.

The wild animals that come to us without injury or serious illness, which might just be suffering from a bit of exposure after a storm or struggling with malnourishment and dehydration, are generally the ones that stand the best chance of pulling through and making a full recovery. Others may be suffering from very minor injuries that can be quickly dealt with, or that may not be incompatible with survival.

One wild bird story that sticks in my mind involved a 'scorrie' brought to us with a damaged leg. A scorrie is what locals call a seagull, usually a herring gull. We gave rudimentary treatment and kept her in our aviary overnight; on reassessment the next day, it was felt that the injury was unlikely to affect her ability to cope in the wild.

We took her down to Scrabster Beach to let her go, opening the cage and allowing her to take flight under her own steam. As she climbed higher into the air, another scorrie flew in from the direction of the sea. It arrived by our patient's side and together they soared high across the bay as a couple. It was quite a romantic sight to behold, almost as if a mate had been waiting, keeping vigil in anticipation of her return. They would have had a lot to catch up on over their fish supper that night, after what must have been a very strange 24 hours for any seabird to have experienced!

One of the more dramatic wildlife stories in recent times involved an infrequent visitor to our shores. It isn't uncommon to hear of cetacean species (large sea mammals) being spotted from our clifftops and beaches, especially in the summer and autumn, when harbour porpoises, bottlenose dolphins, common dolphins and even orcas and minke whales have all been known to make an appearance. But there are other sea mammals that offer only occasional sightings at best; and to have one of those extraordinary creatures alive, and at touching distance, is truly a once-in-a-lifetime experience.

Atlantic white-sided dolphins seldom stray close enough for a clear sighting from land. They far prefer the deeper water, where they feed on dense shoals of squid, mackerel, herring and shrimp. They get their name from the white stripe that runs along their sides before it blends into a light mustard-yellow towards the tail stock. In terms of dolphins, they sit at the larger end of the scale, with males reaching an impressive length of up to nine feet. However, in spite of their association with deep drop-offs and the open sea, an Atlantic white-sided once found itself stranded here in Caithness, on Dunnet Beach.

The phenomenon of whales or dolphins stranding (or beaching) themselves on land is still not wholly understood, and theories as to the cause range from simply the shallow, sloping coastal topography throwing off the echolocation ability of some deeper-water species, to the animal being injured, sick, old or just badly disorientated. It's probably more common than you think; in fact, the Zoological Society of London's Cetacean Strandings Investigation Programme (CSIP) has logged more than 12,000 stranded cetaceans since 1990. There have been several along our coastline involving other species, but to our knowledge, this was the first Atlantic white-sided dolphin, and it was in a very poor state.

Early in the morning, a member of the public discovered the dolphin beached, but alive, and put a call in to the SSPCA and the BDMLR (British Divers Marine Life Rescue), who sent someone out to Dunnet to advise and aid an attempted rescue. Unfortunately, the sea was too rough at Dunnet, so the 2.5-metre-long, 230kg male was lifted onto a trailer via an airbed and then transported 10 miles west to the more sheltered beach at Scrabster.

It is always a race against time to save a beached cetacean of any species. Whales are only able to sustain such a massive weight because of the support the seawater offers their body; but out of the water and on land, without that support, their full body weight will actually crush their organs, reducing circulation and causing deadly toxins to build up in their systems. Dolphins fare a little better on account of their smaller size, and are obviously easier to move with a few helping hands, yet their survival rate from a beaching is still low, especially if they have been out of the water for several hours.

It was thought that the dolphin was likely to be quite dehydrated from its ordeal, and that was when our surgery first became involved. It seems superficially ridiculous that a water-dwelling creature could become dehydrated, but it's a case of 'water, water, everywhere, nor any drop to drink'. Just as we find saltwater makes us more, rather than less, thirsty, cetaceans, too, must replenish their fluids from the food they eat, not the ocean.

Vet Tom was soon on the scene, examining the dolphin before tubing 4 litres of rehydration fluid directly down its throat with a calf feeding tube. Cetaceans breathe through the blowholes on top of their heads, so there isn't huge concern about causing them additional distress by rehydrating them straight down their gullet. Rather counterintuitively, despite the wonderful apparatus for breathing out of the top of their heads, if you just let the tide come back in over a beached cetacean, the seawater can drown the animal via the blowhole before there's enough depth for it to lift itself clear of the beach and swim off.

The dolphin was carried into the water by volunteers and supported to ensure it could breathe normally. Gently, it was rocked back and forth in an effort to regather its bearings. The hope, on release, was that the dolphin would swim out to sea; however, as soon as it was let go it simply turned itself around and swam straight back onto the beach. It was assumed then that there was likely to be a disease or disorder affecting its brain and onboard navigation system – perhaps an infection with the bacterial disease 'brucellosis' – rendering it unable to recognise the difference between the deeper water and the deadly shallows. In short, it seemed very sick indeed.

As hard as everyone tried that day, this magnificent creature was simply showing no signs of being able to rescue itself. After several failed attempts, the dolphin was clearly growing progressively weaker: its breathing rate had elevated alarmingly and it was also flexing in distress. With no options left, the decision was made by the BDMLR to euthanise the animal for the sake of its welfare, and the surgery was called into action again.

You could be forgiven for thinking that this would be a task to be undertaken only by a marine life veterinary specialist, but, as is so often the case in our remote part of the world, when it comes to animal emergencies of any kind, we are usually the only option. We have all grown accustomed to the fact that we may be landed with the responsibility of attending to an unfamiliar species once in a blue moon. We approach these unique jobs with a measured and pragmatic mindset. It may not instil confidence if we admit to frantically dipping into books and internet resources, but you must remember we have great experience of similar problems and procedures in other species, and so just a little research on the relevant anatomy and idiosyncrasies allows for an effective transfer of skills in most cases.

Vet Shondie was on call that day. This would be her first (and likely only) experience of euthanising a dolphin, so, as she travelled to Scrabster, she put in a call to one of our retired vets, Sinclair Manson, for some advice. Sinclair is one of Thurso's old guard and is armed with a wide breadth of knowledge on veterinary medicine and wildlife. Shondie knew he was highly likely to have some useful wisdom to offer. He told Shondie she should first consider sedating it with an injection into its muscle, but recommended a very long needle to penetrate the dolphin's blubber (the thick layer of fat cetaceans have to keep them warm in the sea). Then, for the final injection, he also advised her to try to locate the major vein in the dolphin's fluke – its tail fin.

Down at Scrabster, a small crowd had gathered. There were members of the public in wetsuits trying to help, as well as the SSPCA inspector. Shondie was admittedly nervous as she prepared her equipment, kneeling next to this eight-foot-long sea creature for the very first time, and surrounded by an audience, but she kept her cool and put the pressure from the gallery to one side.

There are always going to be variations and challenges from species to species, but the actual clinical process of putting an animal to sleep is fairly uniform. If an animal is particularly fractious or in distress – as the dolphin was that day, flexing and occasionally thrashing on the beach – we will usually sedate it first. Once Shondie had felt the dolphin was suitably calmed from the sedative she had administered, she reached for the drug we ultimately use for the job of sending the animal into its permanent sleep: a barbiturate called pentobarbital (historically 'pentobarbitone' in the UK, or just 'pentobarb', as we know it).

In reduced doses it can be used as an anaesthetic for veterinary surgery – though it rarely is nowadays – and it may still have certain uses in human medicine. Pentobarbital dampens the 'higher' centres of the brain first, initially resulting in loss of consciousness; but with a greater dose, the more basic regions of the brain start to shut down, causing a cessation in vital functions and resulting in respiratory arrest. Having pentobarb in the bloodstream is not distressing or painful. After intravenous dosing, it starts to take effect in a matter of seconds, and usually within a minute all will have stopped; the animal will have passed away. People must be reassured that any short-lived twitching or gasping is entirely involuntary – remember, the first thing to disappear is consciousness. Our aim is always for the process to be smooth, stressless and pain-free.

Shondie slid the needle into the position advised by Sinclair and, by luck or intuition, successfully hit the vein in the groove of the dolphin's fluke on her first try. She then injected two syringes of pentobarb, and there was no reaction nor any excess stress for the dolphin. Air ceased flowing through its blowhole and it slipped from its suffering quickly and peacefully.

I understand that the euthanasia of cetaceans such as whales can be trickier than with smaller animals. Firstly, if they are still moving, it can be dangerous to be close to the tail and fins. Also, access to blood vessels can become very difficult as animal size increases, and so there is a risk of injecting outside of the vein. Additionally, the volume of pentobarbital required is huge and can be an environmental concern. Indeed, I read a report of a dog who slipped into what appeared to be a coma after chewing an unknown substance on a beach. Thankfully, the dog revived after three days but it was discovered that the substance had been blubber, laced with pentobarb, from a euthanised whale. Other approaches are now being used for whale euthanasia, including into-the-heart injection of safer chemicals, or simple exsanguination (bleeding out) after sedation.

In this member of a smaller species, Shondie confirmed death: listening for its heart with her stethoscope, confirming there was absolutely no air passing in or out of the blowhole, and finally checking the corneal reflex by touching the eyeball to see if a blink was elicited. The final act was to lift the animal onto a low trailer, cover it with a tarpaulin and take it to a safe place overnight. Early the next morning, members of the Scottish Marine Animals Strandings Scheme transported the body to a lab in Inverness for a post-mortem.

For all of the disappointments that came with the death of such a graceful and intelligent marine animal that day, Shondie was right to feel a real professional pride at how smoothly the whole process had gone. In this instance, the dolphin had undoubtedly experienced a better end to its life than it would have if just left to languish miserably on the beach, and sometimes, with wildlife, that's the best outcome you can reasonably hope for.

Chapter Twenty-One

Equine Issues

This is going to sound like I'm stating the blindingly obvious: owning a horse is a significant step-up in expense and commitment from your average household pet. Not only is it an expensive animal to purchase in itself, but there is considerable outlay involved in its keeping. Unless you own your own land, then livery fees will need to be paid. Even if you do own a field or two, shelters, stables and supplementary feeding will be required. Then the farrier will be called upon for shoeing and you'll also need tack (rugs, bridles, saddles); you may even invest in a trailer or transporter to travel to equestrian events. Oh, and of course, there are the vets' fees.

My girls would have had to display a *serious* level of commitment before I even considered getting them their own horse. However, as part of a rich mix of childhood experiences, they took riding lessons when they were young, and they thoroughly enjoyed them. My own experience on horseback, however, leaves a lot to be desired.

Don't get me wrong, I'm very comfortable by the side of a horse with a stethoscope or a needle in hand; as a vet, horses and I understand each other at that level, but sitting on one's back has more than once left me … well, *not* sitting on its back! The most dramatic example of this was on my gap year in Africa. The base camp in the game reserve had stables with horses, and what sounds more idyllic than riding on horseback across the open savannah, the African sun on your back and herds of wildebeest and antelope grazing before you?

I was young, foolhardy and up for a new adventure. I didn't want to admit to having precious little experience on horseback, so I thought I'd let the stableman work that out for himself by watching me make an idiot of myself. My four-hooved escort for the morning was bay, tall and muscular. Even during the simple trot out of base camp, I bounced off the saddle and had to remount. It was a huge horse to fall from, but I couldn't lose face now. I jumped back on and pretended it was nothing. We then entered a large fenced-off area of reserve where my horse spotted one of its pals half a mile away and spontaneously broke into a full gallop.

It is odd what can go through your mind when death is staring you in the face. I managed to think how much easier it was to stay on the horse in a gallop as opposed to the earlier trot. I managed to think how exhilarating it was to be moving at full pelt on horseback. Then I started thinking, *How do I stop it?* I pulled on the reins, but it had no effect at all. I was starting to get scared; the horse didn't seem to care a hoot that there was a useless human on its back.

I don't know whether the stirrup snapped or whether I just decided to bail out of the whole situation. I flew off in an arc through the air at rocket speed and landed with a thud. I lay motionless and dazed for a minute or so until two or three heads with anxious expressions peered at me over the tall African grass, their faces clearly announcing the question foremost in their minds: *Is he still alive?*

I was sore and my ribs creaked as I breathed for a few days. It could so easily have been a fatal fall at that speed. I have been on horseback since and managed to stay in place, but by their side with my veterinary armoury is where I feel most secure!

What do you need to be a horse vet? I read a jocular article once portraying the following stereotypes based on car preference: the farm vet loves a practical pickup truck or a four-wheel drive of some kind. If you're a small-animal vet, you're likely to be found in a family saloon, but it's got to be a fairly high-spec model with a few swish gadgets and features. And then there's the equine vet, swooshing around immaculately in their brand-new Porsche. The stereotype dictates that the equine vet is the Flash Harry of the veterinary world. They've got to look the part as they are sweeping into the stables: impeccably groomed, smelling of money in their fancy car, with a posh watch and a pair of plush designer wellies; they are the profession's cool characters.

Stereotypes can be fun, but many examples of where they hold no water can always be found. On our patch, we all treat horses regularly, but the vet who does the majority of our equine work is Tom. He doesn't drive a sports car, and the last time he was immaculately groomed could well have been his wedding day. Breaking the mould, he's basically a down-to-earth farmer. He is really well liked by our horse-owning clients, though, to such an extent that someone on *The Highland Vet* series even went as far as to say 'every surgery should have a Tom'. I can't recall such a grand statement being broadcast about anyone else in the team, but despite such an accolade there's no point rolling out the red carpet for him at the practice; he would soon soil it with his muddy boots.

In Caithness and north Sutherland we don't have any big racing yards, likely influenced by the fact there are no racecourses this far north, but there are a few people who keep some of the more expensive horses, and others involved in breeding them. The smaller and miniature breeds, such as Shetland ponies, are quite popular among enthusiasts, both for children to ride and as a cute wee companion for other horses. A variety of horse and pony* breeds will be kept for pleasure by people who just love horses. Activities will range from taking a horse out on a 'hack' – a bit of light exercise in the countryside – to travelling to horse shows and competitions.

Horses can get themselves into a host of problems. We will commonly see cuts and wounds; these are occasionally caused by some activity with their owners, but sometimes they seem to spontaneously appear – presumably down to fun and antics with their field-mates. Broken bones are less common, thankfully, as they can lead to euthanasia, although more can be done for fractures nowadays than in former eras. With our glorious coastline, another idyllic scene is that of riding along a beach in the sunset, but I recall once diagnosing a broken bone just above the hoof of a horse that pulled up lame after a good gallop out on the sand. You may think such a surface has a lot of give to it but, in actuality, sand compacting under a rapidly moving hoof might as well

---

* A pony is distinguished from a horse as anything less than 14.2 hands in height. A 'hand' is the traditional unit used to measure horses; originally based on the breadth of a human hand, it's now standardised at 4 inches.

be concrete. Thankfully, smaller bones such as the one this horse broke can be amenable to surgical repair at a specialist centre.

Lameness (limping) without anything as dramatic as a broken bone can be a minefield to diagnose. It is a fairly common presentation, much easier if they are hardly weight-bearing or displaying a clear injury like a swelling or a cut; but when lameness is subtle, figuring out which leg is the lame leg isn't always as straightforward as you'd assume. An owner may perceive a subtle change in motion but not be able to specify why, or a rider could notice something slightly out of kilter while in the saddle. In those cases, vets have to watch the horse closely as it trots up and down. We ask ourselves questions including, 'Are the buttocks moving asymmetrically when it trots away from us?' 'Is the head thrown up minutely as it places one of its front feet when coming towards us?'

Even once you've isolated the lame leg, you still have to try to work out where on the leg the pain resides. As a general rule, I was taught that 90 per cent of lameness cases originate in the foot. As much as it is always best to assume nothing, we at the practice still tend to start our investigations from the foot up. If the foot has been ruled out, we move up the leg and, when necessary, can employ 'flexion tests', where we hold the leg up and flex each of the joints sequentially and individually. Most of you will have suffered a sore joint at some time, perhaps an ankle, and found that if you sit with it in one position for a while or apply tension to it for a short time, then it will be stiff and sorer for a few seconds on moving it again. We utilise this principle by flexing, say, the fetlock joint on the front leg for a minute, then we let the horse go and watch for increased lameness on that leg for the first few steps as it is led away. If present, then the fetlock could be the culprit. If not, we move on to the next joint. Another method to isolate the region of pain is to use 'nerve blocks', where we apply local anaesthetic at strategic points around nerves to block out the sensation to certain parts of the leg or foot. If the horse then trots away sound, you know the lameness is located in whichever part of the leg you've just numbed.

Back to the foot, there can be multiple causes of lameness, but a common and satisfying diagnosis is an abscess. The horse will go rapidly lame, sometimes in as quickly as 24 hours, to the point of only toe-touching or non-weight-bearing. We will examine the foot with 'hoof testers', essentially enormous pliers, and use them to work methodically around the sole, placing direct pressure on certain points until eventually the horse reacts. Once we find the spot, we will dig down into the foot until we strike oil in the form of a sudden squirt of pus as the pressure in the abscess is released. It's not just horses that can suffer from this complaint; recently I drained an abscess from a bull, grinding down into its hoof with power tools until the pus oozed out. It's a very gratifying result for a vet, and a huge relief for the animal.

Laminitis is another common foot condition suffered by horses. The laminae (plural of 'lamina') are the soft tissues that hold the horny hoof wall on to the toe bone within the foot. When this adhesion breaks down, it can be agonising, even leading to rotation of the toe bone within the hoof. There is a fairly complex set of causes, but we often see laminitis in ponies associated with enjoying the seasonally available rich, lush grass. You may notice ponies grazing on quite bare pasture specifically to avoid this problem. Treatment inevitably includes pain-relieving medication and may well involve working with a farrier, a specialist in equine hoof care, who will apply therapeutic shoeing to the affected horse's feet – frequently working together with the vet and using any X-ray images we may have acquired.

Colic is also a typical reason for emergency calls to horses. If you've had children, you are probably more aware of colic; it is not a disease in its own right, but rather the name we give to a present- ing symptom: bellyache. Causes of such abdominal pain are many, and so the level of investigation and types of treatment vary. Whatever the cause, a horse will usually sweat and roll around on the ground in an attempt to relieve its discomfort, before getting back to its feet to pace agitatedly. As vets, we assess pain by moni- toring heart rate, and then we gather other information about the cause of the colic by listening to the gut activity with our stetho- scopes and examining, as for cows, with our arms in the rectum.

Some cases of colic require surgical intervention, and fast. However, we unfortunately cannot offer surgical facilities for horses in our remote location. Yet, transporting a horse many hours to a centre in the south when it is already in a lot of pain and prone to rolling, and when the condition might deteriorate to a point beyond redemption while in transit, would only be appli- cable in a very few cases; the question of the animal's welfare must be raised. For these reasons, I'm sorry to say, 'surgical colic' up here usually ends in euthanasia.

On the bright side, however, there are many cases we can treat medically. 'Spasmodic colic' is a vague working term for hyper- motility of the bowel – gurgly guts, in other words. Through the stethoscope we hear excessive gut activity in the guise of squelches and squeaks, and we usually breathe a sigh of relief, because reduced gut activity is much more of a worry. These cases often settle with time and medication to relieve spasm of the intestinal muscle.

Occasionally we see a colic due to impaction. A horse, like a rabbit, is a hind-gut fermenter and, as such, has a huge large intestine. To fit all this voluminous pipework into its abdomen, the intestine doubles back on itself. The resulting bends are termed 'flexures', and one common sticking point is the pelvic flexure. Faecal material can bung up the colon in this region, preventing anything from moving beyond that blockage. On examination, we might feel the impaction by gentle rectal exploration and then treat with pain relief, lots of oral fluids and possibly lubricants by stomach tube; all this is aimed at softening the impacted material and smoothing its passage. The blockage can take a day or more to shift with repeated treatments, but once again, there is that bizarre – and yet genuine – sense of reward in seeing a large pile of poo behind your patient!

Routine equine work revolves around vaccinations and dental checks. As with humans, a regular check of the teeth is recommended. The common symptom to watch for, if a horse does have problems with its teeth, is 'quidding' – the term used when a horse starts to drop half-chewed food chunks from its mouth. Among other problems, sharp edges can develop on the cheek teeth (chewing teeth), which need to be filed down perhaps once or twice a year. We place a gag or speculum in the horse's mouth to keep it open to examine the oral cavity and then file down these edges. In the past, I have used hand rasps for this, which do the job well, but it can be hard work. Now Tom, perhaps with just a hint of Flash Harry, uses power tools for this task (more often than not, with the horse sedated).

Another reason for a dental check would be if the horse is struggling with its bit, the metal bar that sits in the large gap between the horse's incisors at the front and the cheek teeth further back. The bit is the part of the bridle that a rider uses to control their horse's head. In the first series of *The Highland Vet*, a young horse was found to have 'wolf teeth', a pair of small teeth residing at the back of the gap where the bit sits. Not all horses have these teeth, and they're considered vestigial (diminished in form, with no useful purpose); it is suggested that ancient equines would have foraged far tougher foods than those of today and would have used the wolf teeth to split and crush twigs and rough shrubs for their sustenance. They don't always need to be removed, but if interfering with the bit, they can be extracted with no detriment to the horse.

No matter what ailment has caused the horse to require the services of a vet, there is one thing that unites nearly all horses: they are big, they are strong and they have an exceptionally powerful kick. Whether or not horse vets live up to the reputation of being cool and flash, perhaps they do deserve some respect; after all, a published study has found that being an equine vet carries a very high risk of injury. A third of the injuries reported required hospital admission, while 7 per cent involved loss of consciousness.

As I've previously explained, we will hold cows in a crate (or 'crush') designed to restrain them safely. By contrast, a horse is of similar size and weight and possesses a potentially higher capacity to injure humans, yet all too often it is presented with a sole person holding a rope tied to its head collar. Said person may well inform the vet what a well-behaved sweetie pie the horse is, but, of course, it always is for the hand that feeds and grooms it; don't forget we're 'the enemy' armed with a needle! Incidentally, this is paralleled in the comment 'He doesn't bite' from dog owners, which experience has taught us to interpret with caution!

(Numerous owners know exactly how their horse, or dog, will react to the vet and so they willingly forewarn us; and we really appreciate that. In fact, a client at the surgery just the other day kindly warned a young vet about to examine their cat, 'He doesn't like you.' However, the vet was stuck for a response when the owner followed this up by admitting, 'And I don't particularly like you either.' It appears we need thick skin to defend ourselves from more than just teeth and claws!)

Many horses are lovely and well mannered, or at least manageable, but if a horse decides to literally kick off there is very little anyone can do to stop it, and that's when the risk of a serious injury is at its utmost. There are cattle crush equivalents for horses, called 'stocks', which certainly help restrict their movements, but only the biggest of equestrian facilities will have such items. Sedating the animal can help, of course. Mind you, just achieving that still means getting a needle into their neck to inject the sedative, which is no mean feat if they are stomping around, bucking and desperate to get away from the nasty vet. Telling animals, 'It's for your own good' (which I do find myself saying) just never seems to work!

I've been fortunate enough to never have been significantly injured by a horse, but I've certainly had to evacuate a stable or two at a rapid pace. And one of the lecturers at university in my day was right on the verge of retirement when he was kicked in the head by a horse, and subsequently lost an eye. But the worst injury to happen to any of the Thurso vets was, you guessed it, to Ken.

Ken was down at the local college, demonstrating to equestrian students exactly how to sedate a horse, when it happened. He was, in his own words, a fresh 23-year-old vet keen to show off his skills to a youthful audience. Poor Ken. He was presented with a horse notorious for being cantankerous at the very best of times. As he advanced with needle in hand, the horse immediately reared up, kicked out a hoof and knocked him clean out. The concussion was so bad, the course leader had to give him mouth-to-mouth resuscitation in front of the students until eventually an ambulance arrived and carried him off to hospital.

Luckily, he made a full recovery and was back to work a couple of days later; but salt was definitely rubbed into his wound when he attended that year's county show. To his horror, his nemesis was declared the 'Champion of Champions'.

I hope these cautionary tales don't put any of you readers off, especially if you may be considering entering the veterinary profession or even just working with horses. Accidents are rare, especially the bad ones, and many may be avoidable if we take the time to think about our approach. So many of us that have been injured in our work can look back and think of things we could have done differently, and, as we all gather that knowledge and experience and pass it on to the next generation, the job will hopefully get safer year-on-year.

There are, unfortunately, those injuries that are just plain bad luck, and a case of 'wrong place, wrong time', but I hope that you can see there is still an overwhelming amount of reward and satisfaction on offer too. Of course, your level of risk can always be mitigated to a degree, even when working with horses. In spite of all the suave stereotypes bandied about when we humble mixed-practice vets consider the horse specialist, many years ago I heard of an equine vet further south who ditched all pretence of 'cool' and simply started turning up for his jobs with a helmet and full visor. Considering such protective equipment is now encouraged for all working with horses, not just those on their backs – I think that says it all!

Chapter Twenty-Two

A Horse in the Strath

It had been a long, hard day in the surgery. I was first on call and my day shift had merged seamlessly with my night shift as I attended to a poorly dog that had come to us as the standard working hours came to an end. As it approached 8pm I was finishing off and looking forward to getting home. I was starving. Of course, we have a stash of food at the clinic for emergencies, and by that I mean human nutritional 'emergencies'. These generally arise on the back of animal emergencies or just a downright heavy workload. The sweetie tub or biscuit tin, in my opinion, is as essential a part of any vet's kit as their overalls or calving ropes. For example, at 2am, as staff are mustered to help with a bitch caesarean section, a sugar rush, however unhealthy it may be, can help maintain spirits and focus. But that evening I was trying to be well behaved. I knew dinner was waiting and so I virtuously abstained. Then the phone rang.

It was bad enough that the call was to a horse with a big wound on its shoulder, but I may have unintentionally verbalised my feeling of shock when I was informed where the horse currently resided. Achentoul is remote, a long drive from Thurso. Not that a call to that location is fundamentally an unpleasant experience – in fact, quite the opposite. Heading west out of Caithness into the northern portion of our neighbouring county of Sutherland is, in my opinion, one of the perks of the job. The countryside becomes more rugged, the human population becomes more sparse and even the accent is discernibly different to those with an ear for such things. I just love it. A 'west call', like any other call, may lead to a task ranging from cushy to grotty, but unless it's dark or dreich, or both, then the drive can more than make up for anything that may await you.

Rolling over the hill beyond the small village of Reay, the vast expanse of this bleak but strangely appealing county opens up before you as you make your way west along the north coast. On a clear day, with a nice wee job awaiting me, and perhaps even a cup of tea, I have often thought incredulously, *I'm getting paid for this!* Similarly, as the North Coast 500 route has brought more and more tourists to appreciate this part of the world, I watch the camper vans pass fleetingly through the scenery and smugly think to myself, *This is my patch, I come here frequently.*

This evening, however, I had mixed feelings. Such a call may be a dream during the working day, and even at this time I was guaranteed a pleasant drive into Sutherland as the sun was setting, yet it was a distant call that would take hours and see me arrive back in the dark. Oh, and did I mention I was starving?

I gathered a pile of equipment and meds that I thought might be required on top of the kit I kept in my car. This was not a call to arrive at to discover I didn't have something critical; there would be no nipping back to the surgery for anything once

I was there. I diverted the phones, as usual, to my home and called Jennifer to explain the situation. Always caring about my well-being in these circumstances (which is reassuring in a wife, I feel), she tried to persuade me to come home quickly for some food. Normally I decline as I just want to get on with the job, or perhaps the nature of the call is too much of an emergency, but on this occasion, I accepted the offer. (On a more general note, knowing how much of an emergency any one call will be is something that comes with experience; calls vary in level of urgency. Often, when faced with several calls, we must triage to varying degrees; if in doubt, where we can, we get there as soon as possible. On this occasion, a few minutes' delay would not be significant, and I figured the horse would benefit from me having been nourished; I would mentally and physically be in a better state to treat her.)

I swung past home, where Jennifer was microwaving my dinner that had been fresh a couple of hours ago. I threw it down my throat like a starved caveman. I didn't enjoy it, and Jennifer has long since stopped being offended on such occasions. Ingesting cold or reheated food and eating at great speed are skills all vets who provide an on-call service are wise to develop early on in their careers. I remember, in a former job as a young vet, being invited to my boss's house for a meal. Neither of us were on call – it was a social evening with opportunity to relax and savour the repast – yet my boss polished off his food at great speed. His wife felt the need to apologise on his behalf, and she enquired of Jennifer as to whether I did the same. The seeming gluttony was put down to the principle 'Eat while you have the chance'. Such is the life of a vet on call.

I left the edge of town, heading west along the main coastal road. It was a very pleasant evening. The light cloud cover in the sky ahead of me diffused the glow of the low sun into a variegated display of orange hues. Having resigned myself to the necessity of this long-distance call, and despite the mild nag of uncertainty at what I would be faced with on arrival, I felt a sense of ease knowing that there were far worse hands I could have been dealt. After the village of Reay, I had to turn away from the sunset and drive perpendicular to the north coast, following Strath Halladale southwards. ('Strath', like 'glen', is a Scottish word for a 'valley'.)

In an upstream direction, I flanked the river that meanders to the sea from the depths of the inland expanse of open moorland. I was blissfully 'roaming in the gloaming' on the single-track road that runs the length of the strath as I cut through a wider region of the Flow Country that extends into much of northern Sutherland and sweeps towards the mountains in the west. I passed the charming and unassuming crofts that line the narrow road, many of which evoked memories: that building on the left was where crofter Donny was knocked over and fell flat on his nose when we were dehorning his neighbour's calves several years ago; for a long couple of seconds I was worried he might never stand up again. Then, by the cemetery on the right, was where I spent hours chasing Alasdair's cow in the snow one winter's morning until, eventually, we managed to pen her up in another crofter's barn to relieve her womb of its calf.

I weaved my way south along the strath as the evening glow slowly faded. Beyond Forsinard there was still enough daylight to appreciate the stunning scenery as it unfolded around me. I was enjoying the music my phone was streaming to my car stereo system, the remote and ancient hills sitting in stark juxtaposition to the fact that, out here in the middle of nowhere, I was flying down a single-track road and streaming data in a man-made bubble!

This journey itself couldn't be more different than the first time I was called to Achentoul. In my early days working in the Highlands, I was called here to help a cow giving birth with its calf stuck halfway out – not really an ideal situation for the calf when a vet has so far to travel. Perhaps its reluctance to enter the world was based on the weather it was sensing outside. It was an awful night; particularly at the top of the strath, the car was beaten by wind and lashing rain. I had already visited crofts in the northern portion of the strath as part of my daywork, but I was now to go beyond them in the storm and the dark into what was, for me at least, unchartered territory. In an era that pre-dated routine GPS in vehicles, I had no idea how far to travel or what I was looking for. I just kept driving and driving, with only ghostly forms of the landscape visible around me; just the occasional building or crop of trees provided reassurance that I wasn't on a causeway across the dark side of the moon. In the end, though, the sparsity of dwellings actually made finding my patient relatively easy; it was a case of *Just head for the light*. I made the assumption I had arrived when, after a long stretch of darkness, a lit-up farm building came into view by a small group of old houses.

This evening, however, almost an hour after leaving Thurso, I approached Achentoul in much more favourable climatic conditions. I pulled up outside the stable where Heather was waiting with her horse, Kari. Darkness was falling quickly by now and as I walked inside, the electric light illuminated a huge, deep gash near Kari's left shoulder. As mentioned, horses with cuts here and there on their bodies, particularly limbs, are a common part of an equine vet's workload, but this was a whopper. It wasn't so much the length – perhaps six inches – but the depth! How on earth had she injured herself in this way? The wound was gaping widely, and I was concerned that tissue tensions would prevent surgical closure, or if I did get it together, that it would burst open again within a few days.

With a gloved hand I explored the area. Kari was remarkably calm about the whole thing; bizarrely, she was bearing weight almost normally and permitted gentle probing of the wound. There is a lot of muscle coverage in this area, high up on a horse's forelimb, and as I examined the cut, my fingers disappeared beyond my second knuckle joint. It was deep! Heather squirmed and said she didn't know how I could do that; she could barely look at it.

For any further examination and treatment, I was best to sedate Kari and numb the area, both for her sake and for mine, if I wished her to remain comfortable and compliant as I tried to piece her back together.

I requested fresh warm water and retrieved sedative drugs from my car. The intravenous injection had the desired effect; Kari's head started to hang. We rarely need horses fully anaesthetised for such procedures. Indeed, in a field setting a full general anaesthetic, by necessity, has to be very limited; longer procedures require full equine hospital facilities. A horse can only be kept anaesthetised for a short period without measures in place to counter what occurs in a recumbent animal. Gravity exerts a significant effect on the circulation, and when the animal is lying on one side, fluid accumulates in the lower lung. Such 'hypostatic congestion' will cause respiratory challenges for the patient. The larger the animal, the more significant the problem, so whereas we rarely need to consider it in cats and dogs, lung congestion is a real concern in horses and other large species. Thus, for many procedures such as this, we use 'standing chemical restraint' – we immobilise the horse but keep it standing. I also infiltrated local anaesthetic around the wound to desensitise the area as best I could.

I then probed the wound again, and as my hand disappeared deep into the muscle, I could feel just a very thin layer of soft tissue remaining over the bone surface of the humerus. The shoulder joint was also very close by. The big worry for a horse, or any species for that matter, is the penetration of a joint space. Contamination leading to infection in a joint is perilous. It could result in euthanasia, or at best a prolonged course of treatment that may still leave the animal with some loss of function. I probed with my fingers, desperately hoping to find no evidence that the wound extended into the joint. I convinced myself we were in the clear, so now for the tricky task of somehow piecing the muscle and skin back together.

With a splash of disinfectant in the water and a huge syringe designed for feeding lambs via a stomach tube, I flushed and flushed the wound to remove as much contamination as possible. Heather commented that she was consoled that it was I who was stitching her horse, as she'd heard that it would therefore be a neat job. Of course, everyone feels a warm glow when affirmed in such a way, but I have learnt to temper any such flattery with realism. On one hand, the comment was welcome at 10pm after a long day; it was reassuring to know that the client had faith in the vet attending to her precious horse. On the other hand, not wishing to be set up for a fall, I felt the need to explain all the possible complications and challenges that may ensue from here on. It was a fact that such a significant wound was unlikely to heal up uneventfully; in the days or even weeks to follow, I fully expected partial or even substantial wound breakdown, along with some discharge and the need for re-examination or possibly revision surgery.

I opened my sterile operating kit and worked at pulling the muscle together as quickly as possible. It wasn't the most satisfying stitch-up. Due to being made of bundles of fibres, muscle is not the easiest tissue to suture, especially when severed across those fibres (sutures with any tension are prone to cutting through the muscle tissue like cheese wire). On top of this, the muscle edges were tattered, but I managed to pull bits together and close some of the dead space – one of the principles of surgery I remember being taught many years ago at vet school.

The skin edges aligned more satisfactorily; still, comments of how well it had come together didn't allay my fears that complications in healing were extremely likely. I was fighting the clock as I put in the final stitches – the sedation was beginning to lighten. I cleaned up the area and dosed Kari with antibiotics and anti-inflammatories. *A job well done ... at least for now,* I thought.

I left medication for administration in Kari's food, gathered my stuff into my car and bade farewell. The long drive back up the strath in the dark was not totally without interest. A few minutes up the road, what looked like the form of a reindeer crossed in front of me. It seemed incongruously out of season; Christmas was still some time away. The lack of a glowing red nose should have helped more rapid recognition. It was obviously a red deer, the antlers appearing thicker and reindeer-like due to being in velvet. Then, towards the north of the strath, it was the rabbits that darted in and out of the headlights' beam. It must have been about 11pm as I rolled into Thurso. I wondered how well Kari's wound would heal and how soon we would need to attend to her again.

I telephoned the next day to see how things were. The wound was still holding together but Kari was sore. I had left pain relief for her; we discussed doses.

I made contact again a few weeks later when curiosity had got the better of me. I was aware that a little telephoned advice had been sought in the interim, which vet Eilidh had provided. Heather said Kari was doing very well and the wound was on its way to being fully healed, although we both acknowledged that a significant scar would always remain visible. I had been on holiday in the meantime and what I hadn't been aware of was that vet Margaret had been back to review the wound after it had started to gape a little. As I have said, this didn't surprise me in the least. However, Heather said the breakdown hadn't occurred for a full week after surgery, which appeared to have been sufficient time for much of the muscle to knit together. So, when the skin had opened again, there was obvious filling of the gap underneath.

Heather had then braved her reluctance to look at the wound and irrigated it copiously each day, and now just the surface was left to heal over. I was also informed that the tell-tale signs of blood and hair had been found on a projection from a metal gate in Kari's field. The assumption was that some fun and frolics with her companion had got a little out of hand.

Chapter Twenty-Three

All Hallows' Eve

Autumn draws to a close and the nights are drawing in. At first, the failing light is almost imperceptible, but as October flows forward it is undeniable that winter is waiting in the wings. The last Sunday of the tenth month sees an hour stolen back on the clock, and we're soon to be back to rising and returning home in the darkness.

October 31st is, of course, Halloween. It's not an event I get excited about. I have no veterinary ghost stories, but there have been a few harrowing moments during my career – several of them have been retold in these pages. There's been a fair bit of blood and gore too, as well as creatures that are known to get the pulses of some people racing on sight alone.

One such creature was so huge, it was brought to the practice in a box on wheels. Writhing within was a 16-foot python (okay, that's another figure that grows each time I tell it). It was so strong that I conscripted Ken to hold its head while the owner coped with its considerable coils. It had a suspected case of mouth rot – an infection that eats away at the oral cavity. Ken alleges I made him open the mouth while I stood at some distance and examined it with binoculars. I claim no recollection of such cowardice.

What I do remember, however, was the owner's suggestion when he wanted to put the snake back in its box: 'You should step away. You've annoyed him, so he might go for you.' Needless to say, I did retreat at that point and left the room for a minute!

I do also recall questioning the sanity of a client when he brought in a snake for an X-ray one day. Wearing a maniacal grin, he said, 'Watch this,' and proceeded to deliberately waft his hand in front of his legless pet to encourage it to bite him. So it did.

There are also those moments that fall outside the conventions of plain scary or harrowing and into a category purely of their own. These are the incidents that are utterly unique – the experiences that will remain vividly in our memories for many years to come and require no embellishment in order to stand alone as fabulous tales. One such occasion came one late autumn's evening, and it will surprise no one by now to discover that Ken was involved too.

Brian was a shy, reclusive older gentleman with a dog called Sula. His lone bungalow sat by a road out towards John O'Groats in quite an exposed, windswept and sparsely populated neck of the county. We would always visit his home to treat his pets.

The sad day arrived, as it does for all pets, when Brian knew 'the time had come'. Poor old Sula was nearing the end and, as much as he wanted to hold on to her for his own sake, he couldn't see her suffer. Brian contacted the surgery one Saturday, and I arranged to make the sorrowful final visit to Sula later that afternoon. Often, we try to take an extra pair of hands to a home euthanasia, just to help everything run smoothly. It was November. Ken and I were on duty that weekend, and the workload had kept us occupied during the morning but had tailed off towards the end of the day, allowing us to go together.

I pulled up my car outside Brian's gate just as the light was beginning to fade from the sky. We knocked and were surprised to be greeted by a lady in uniform. She explained she was the district nurse who had been attending to Brian's medical needs. On hearing of the distressing event that would be occurring, and on sensing his upset, she had offered to stay with him beyond her usual finishing time. A familiar face to help comfort him in his time of need. *What a kind and lovely person,* I thought.

There was a warm glow of electric lighting as we entered the kitchen. To the left stood a small table covered in a sizeable cactus collection and a small box from which emanated soft and soothing birdsong. *'Tweet, tweet, tweet.'* The gadget was designed as a de-stressor, to be played in the background to help people relax. Never a more appropriate time for it than then.

I approached Sula as she lay at Brian's feet and patted her head. The time to say goodbye had come, and I was so glad the nurse had stayed with Brian for moral support. He explained, too, that a man who came regularly to do his garden had dug a grave ready to receive his beloved companion. I got my syringe prepared and, with Ken holding Sula's leg to raise the vein, I let her slip away.

A saddening tale that is all too familiar to pet owners up and down the country. But then, this story took a turn that might, in a way, have been a blessing to distract Brian from his inevitable grief.

Night had now fully fallen and, as Brian was physically going to struggle at any time, we offered to take Sula out to her grave; it was the least we could do. I sent Ken on a reconnaissance mission into the garden to find where the gardener had been digging. It was pretty dark by now and we were out in the countryside with no supplementary lighting, so he strapped on his head torch. Like a miner investigating an unknown pit, he ventured out into the darkness, leaving me chatting and consoling.

A few minutes later Ken returned. 'I've found it,' he announced. Brian made it clear he wanted to be there, so we all made our way outside. Ken illuminated our path with his head torch, holding Sula in his arms. We took it slowly for Brian's sake; he shuffled along behind Ken. The nurse was next, and I followed at the rear of this stately and solemn procession. We made our way around the house and then along to the far corner of the garden, led by our guiding light to Sula's place of rest. The interment ceremony was brief – it was cold and a little blowy – and so, after Ken had shovelled a little soil into place, we all turned and made our way back around the house to the bright patch created by the light over the front door.

But there was a problem: the door had closed on the latch behind us as we had left, and we were trapped out in the cold. 'Oh, I didn't bring a key,' admitted Brian. The nurse began to look a little stressed. Her bag and car keys were inside, and she'd stayed well beyond the call of duty out of the goodness of her heart; how was this now a fair and fitting turn of events? The evening had been tragic enough, but now, with only the light we were under and that of Ken's head torch, we were all stranded in the middle of nowhere in the increasingly chilly Caithness night air.

We stared at each other for a few short moments, then Ken and I had the same idea: 'I wonder if there are any windows open?' I sent Ken around the house for a third time with his faithful head torch. In the meantime, I looked at the windows nearby. There was one into the kitchen on a wall at a right angle to the front door. It comprised the common set-up of a large lower fixed pane plus a small, thin casement section at the top with a multi-holed lever arm so it could be fixed open by varying degrees. I looked at the opening section. A thin, agile person might just fit through that gap. However, the window was closed and fastened on the inside.

I gripped the window frame's lower edge and tried waggling it. To my surprise it was slightly loose, but would I get enough movement to flip the retaining arm up on the inside? I waggled and waggled more vigorously and then, abruptly, the arm sprang up and released. The window was open! But how was I going to get through it?

I climbed precariously onto the narrow window ledge and stuck my head through the small opening. I started pulling myself up and through; I'm not a hefty chap and was slightly thinner back in those days, but I filled the gap. Ken has a larger frame than I, and, by his own later admission, this would not have been an option for him.

As I was hanging, waist folded over the lower edge of the window frame, I had the realisation that manoeuvring through this opening as I might through a larger one was not going to be possible. Ideally, I wanted to step through it or at least redirect myself so that I could land on my feet; but it soon became only too apparent that there was no option but for me to fall from the window and dive head first into the kitchen with precious little control.

Suddenly I felt something grip both my ankles. It was Ken; he had returned without reward from his third torch-lit mission to the back of the house. My body was tight within the window aperture, and Ken started forcefully feeding me inside inch by inch like a postman persuading an oversized package through a high letterbox.

Once my centre of gravity resided more in the kitchen than out, I knew I had reached the point of no return. Soon Ken was supporting my weight as I dangled from his firm hold on my ankles, but at some point, he would have to let go and then I would be set for a rapid headlong descent. Surely this predicament couldn't become more treacherous? But then, I saw what lay in wait beneath me: Brian's cactus collection.

'Tweet, tweet, tweet.' The soothing sound that surrounded the portion of my body now within the house was not having the desired impact on my anxiety level.

At this point in the Hollywood version, *Highland Vet: The Movie*, one of two things would happen depending on the genre of film ultimately desired by the producers. In the serious spy thriller, the tweeting would fade into the *Mission: Impossible* theme tune; Tom Cruise (who would be called upon to play me, of course) would elegantly flip like a trapeze artist in mid-air, land into a smooth forward roll and then coolly find his feet, ready to continue his adventure.

In an equally valid but more comedic production, you would hear a loud 'Aaargh!' as my stunt double plummeted from the window, followed by an immediate cut to a scene of the star – perhaps Rowan Atkinson – sitting dazed against the wall with cactus spines sticking out of his forehead. As it was, I opted to forgo my Academy Award and did neither. Ken, largely making his own decisions from the outside, gave one last shove and let go. In an improvised and unrefined motion, I directed my dive to one side, narrowly missed the cactus table and crumpled inelegantly in a heap on the kitchen floor.

'Tweet, tweet, tweet.' The birds were laughing at me. But who cares? I had done it! I was in.

It did leave me with concerns about the security of Brian's house; I was no professional housebreaker and yet I had managed to sneak my way in. I also realise, on account of this tale, I have now opened myself up to a visit from the local police if ever there is a spate of cat burglaries in Thurso.

With a smile of satisfaction on my face, I walked proudly to the front door and let the others in from the cold. I can still hear Brian standing there repeating, 'That was amazing, that was amazing!' as the birds welcomed him home: *'Tweet, tweet, tweet.'*

Winter

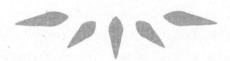

Chapter Twenty-Four

Gunpowder, Treason and Terrified Dogs

I have noticed that the transition from autumn to winter is often so abruptly marked, it can feel like a seasonal switch has been flicked somewhere overnight. All it takes is for one late autumnal storm to arrive just when the trees' leaves are right at their most willing to fall. The wind will strip the branches entirely, and those golden colours of the season are instantly wiped away; what's left behind is the skeletal frame of the naked tree: the stark sign that our coldest season is upon us once again.

We can get some terrific storms throughout early winter. We all know that a tempest with a title bestowed by the Met Office means all of us in the UK are in for a battering, but this can be a blustery and windswept corner of the world even in the absence of a storm with a name. Today is a classic example; it is *wild* outside, so we chose to walk the dog in the shelter of the forest, but not before detouring to the seafront to see the amazing waves and spume. I got out of the car to take a video and was blown off balance. Spectacular!

Thurso has been built to withstand bad weather, but nonetheless, the older Victorian quarters of the town can only bear so much. We had to undertake some fairly major renovations and repairs to our own home after a particularly severe November storm. That round of weather might not have caused much damage in itself, but it certainly helped reveal the scale of the long-term climatological wear and tear to our property, after decades of winter weather had cumulatively compromised the masonry, the pointing and our roof. Leaks were simultaneously revealed in all but one room of our house, with a major area of ingress occurring in the gable via the stones in our chimneys – which, we discovered, were actually just crumbling away to powder. It cost a fortune to repair it all: we had to have the chimney stacks rebuilt, replace the roof slates, and add a protective layer of lime rendering to much of the stonework. But, hopefully, our home will now stay standing for another century or so.

The first frosts generally arrive in November, with that aforementioned climatic lag that occurs between our coastal town and the interior ensuring the ground can often be frozen bullet-hard around the farms and fields well before we see our first dusting of dawn ice out on the lawns of Thurso.

A cold winter's night with a sky clear of clouds can very occasionally offer an opportunity to spot the aurora borealis, perhaps better known as the northern lights (or the 'mirrie dancers', as this natural spectacle is called in Shetland). A quick internet search for the northern lights will bring up thousands of truly spellbinding images and videos of dancing curtains of shimmering light, with magnificent waves of mainly green but also pink, violet and other colours. The phenomenon can be seen in the night skies of both the extreme north and south of the earth's hemispheres (though in the south it goes by the name aurora australis). It's caused by huge clouds of electrically charged particles, originally released by violent storms on the surface of the sun. The particles travel almost 100 million miles before they eventually collide with the earth and either bounce back into space or become trapped in our planet's magnetic field. Once here, they are pulled towards the magnetic north and south poles, where they strike atoms and molecules in our atmosphere, exciting them and facilitating emission of the different colours and creating this famously entrancing mantle of light.

Given Thurso lies at almost the same latitude as the southern tip of Greenland, the Highlands have become something of a destination for people hoping to see the northern lights for themselves. However, seeing these lights in Scotland is far from guaranteed; ideally you need a clear night, very low levels of light pollution and a recent surge of solar surface activity. Even then, if you are lucky enough to see something, don't be too disappointed if it doesn't resemble the stunning images that are captured closer to, and within, the Arctic Circle. Nevertheless, friends of ours have seen nature's light show on numerous occasions, not least because they are optimally positioned on a hillside out of town, with a large picture window looking right out across Thurso Bay and north towards the Orkney Islands.

Often, they'd tell us excitedly, 'Oh, the northern lights were great last night! You should've seen them!' To which we'd think, *Thanks for telling us now, but we needed to know last night!* There are websites that will tell you when the northern lights are likely to display in our area, but rather than rely on anything high-tech like that, we just asked our friends to let us know the next time they saw lights start to appear. Sure enough, one winter's evening we were out walking the dog in the park with town lights and buildings around us when my phone rang with the news that the sky was beginning to glow.

We rushed home, dropped off the dog and elected to get in the car and drive to a point away from any of our small town's light pollution. Anticipation was building – that night, even from our own back garden we were able to see a greenish glowing fuzziness starting to smear its way across the sky. However, in just the few minutes it took us to get to a layby high above the town, the lights had already started to fade. To make matters worse, as we gazed out into the darkness, taking in what was left of the green glow, an elderly lady pulled in beside us and vacated her car to stare into the atmosphere, evidently with the same goal as us. Quite bizarrely, having left behind the glare of the town, she elected to leave her headlights on. There was little point in making a fuss; the opportunity had passed.

There will be future occasions, I know. In fact, I have wondered, when driving out on a call in the small hours, whether I have caught a vague hint of the same spectacle above me. On considering that, I realise that an avid aurora chaser, prepared to endure regular sleepless vigils, will no doubt prove the point that the northern lights are on show at this latitude far more often than I imagine. It's just that I prefer to sleep while they're dancing the night away.

There is a period when spectacular lights in the night sky can be a feast for both eyes and ears. Bonfire Night in Britain famously commemorates the events of the 5th of November 1605, when Guy Fawkes was arrested while guarding a pile of explosives hidden beneath the House of Lords. The intention of Mr Fawkes and his revolutionary band of Catholics was to assassinate King James I, a Protestant, at the State Opening of Parliament. Guy Fawkes was later tortured to the point of confession, implicating his co-conspirators, before they were all condemned to death in a brutal public execution.

A later act of Parliament introduced an annual day of thanksgiving for the survival of the King, encouraging the lighting of bonfires. In the 400 or so years since that fateful evening in the bowels of the House of Lords, the event has long since evolved into quite a merry social occasion. Today, the bonfires might remain, but the night is probably best known for the widespread use of fireworks in anything from large organised and ticketed displays for the public, right down to your neighbour who might have bought a small box of rockets and sparklers for the garden.

My birthday is close to Bonfire Night, so as a young lad I always looked forward to that time of year, with my own party and gifts. Other outings to bonfires and fireworks – with all the associated treats, sparklers and sticky bonfire toffee – would just add to the excitement. Today, though, I have to confess, I'm not so much a fan of either being reminded I'm another year older or all the loud bangs that come along with Bonfire Night. That's not to say I don't still enjoy it all. In recent years, we've been invited to a friend's penthouse flat, which conveniently overlooks Thurso town and the large organised display put on for the community by the local Rotary club down towards the harbour. That, for me, is the perfect way to enjoy the fireworks: sat in the warmth with our friends, some food and a glass of wine to see the sky decorated by a cloudburst of light explosions, without really being able to hear them. It used to be said – unfairly, I think – that children should ideally be seen and not heard; my preference is that the adage be updated to pertain to fireworks!

Given that a firework is essentially an explosive, I do accept that removing the bang altogether will probably prove impossible by the laws of physics, but there is a range of fireworks on the market that are considerably quieter; good news for people like me, and even better news for dogs and other noise-phobic animals, which can include cats, small pets such as rabbits and guinea pigs, and even horses and donkeys.

The distress caused to dogs during the fireworks season should not be underestimated. In fact, according to the Kennel Club, recent research reported that three-quarters of dog owners noticed a 'significant change' in their dog's mood and behaviour during Bonfire Night, and a third of people said that their animal was 'visibly terrified' of fireworks. The Kennel Club also found that the number of dogs that go missing doubles during the fireworks season, with some animals scared so witless, they will even force their way from the home or garden and run in a state of such extreme panic that they are often found cowering many miles away.

Compared to us, dogs can hear sounds at a significantly higher frequency, sounds we are simply unaware of. Their hearing is much more acute too; they're able to detect noise possibly over four times further away than we can. This means that a noise that sounds loud, but tolerable, to you – like a firework in the sky – will seem so much louder to a dog. You might notice your dog becomes agitated (barking, pacing, on edge or panting, with its ears pricked) even when you can't hear the noise of the fireworks yourself from within your living room. For some animals, just a distant 'pop' or even the muted 'ssssssssh' sound of a firework being launched is enough to evoke their fight-or-flight response and bring on enormously high levels of anxiety.

You can't reason with a dog and explain it's nothing to get stressed about. To them it is a very loud alien noise that is both unpredictable and inescapable – although they try to flee if they have the opportunity. Even their supposed safe haven, their home, is violated by the petrifying percussion. If your dog has had a bad response to fireworks in the past, it will not only happen again but it is likely the severity of the phobia will worsen over time. More than that, dogs will make associations very quickly and can work out that the shorter days mean stress is soon to come. They might refuse to go out after dark (which is hard to avoid in November!) or at least be on edge and not fully enjoy their exercise.

Our retriever Fyrish used to suffer really badly during the fireworks season, in which I also include New Year's Eve. I remember one Hogmanay, the expected flurry of fireworks had burst in the sky at midnight. No more were anticipated, so on the evening of New Year's Day we had left Fyrish at home. She was usually quite content with her own company for a period, and we were due to visit my parents to celebrate my dad's birthday.

My parents followed us to Thurso all those years ago. Although they would admit, in truth, they followed their granddaughter; Jennifer and I were a bonus! Additionally, when I was still only a schoolboy, my mum was dismayed that my dad opted not to accept a job offer on Orkney, so the opportunity to move within sight of the islands made for a win-win situation. Ironically, my dad worked much of the last decade of his career on Orkney and loved it!

My parents' house was only a short distance across town. From their lounge I noticed a few fireworks popping in the sky, but I convinced myself they were emerging from a location well away from our own property. However, on returning home, Fyrish didn't greet us at the door as usual, which was a little odd. We flicked on the kitchen light and were shocked to discover she had totally shredded her way through the vinyl flooring by the back door in a desperate attempt to dig her way out of the house. In her mind, consumed by irrational panic, the house was under attack, and her best hope was to escape; she hadn't realised, of course, that had she been successful, she would have actually been more exposed to the noise that terrified her.

We searched every room for Fyrish before we eventually found her. She had squeezed herself behind the spare bed and was cowering in the darkness, hard up against the back wall. Poor thing, she was near inconsolable. I remember, too, it was another New Year's Eve when fireworks were going off well into the small hours that we bent our own house rules and allowed Fyrish to sleep on the bed with us.

Every year, we get people coming into the practice asking what can be done to help their animal cope during the fireworks season. Unfortunately, there is no quick and easy solution, and inevitably many only think about it when it is already too close to the occasion. In these instances, there are some stopgap medications that we can prescribe to help a dog, basically, 'chill out'.

Other solutions are preferable, but they take effort and forethought. Approaching the problem with a bit of doggy psychology, for instance, is a more satisfying strategy because it will help the dog cope in other situations if they are of a naturally nervous disposition and have a tendency towards anxiety and wariness. I recommend speaking to an accredited behaviourist to help you instil confidence and optimism in your dog so that they cope better with novel noises and situations. Most of this is done through games, so your dog should love it. There are also albums and playlists of scary noises available for purchase that can help expose your dog to common sounds in a controlled way and habituate them to all sorts of potential stressors, such as motorbikes, trains and, of course, fireworks. I would recommend using these with puppies during feeding and playtime as part of a rich socialisation programme in those critical early weeks and months.

On Bonfire Night itself, I suggest putting on the television or stereo as background noise and battening down the hatches: close the curtains to avoid visual stimulation from the sky and keep the cat indoors and lock the cat flap. For dogs, it may also help to provide a preoccupying calming activity like munching on an irresistible, tasty chew. Oh, and stay calm yourself or your dog will pick up on your anxiety; by all means, feel free to lie on the rug, chewing on something too. Better still, what we've found to be by far the easiest way of guaranteeing that our dogs don't get too distressed is to take them to stay with our friends who live outside of town for the evening. However, that doesn't help curb their anxiety for the rest of the season; we can't send Milis to our friends from mid-October to January 1st every year. What would be ideal is to know when any fireworks are likely to be set off so that we can work around those specific occasions.

The big display in town is a known and publicised event, so we pet owners can work with that. But smaller private garden parties just happen, and dog owners have no time to react. They can occur randomly for days before and after November 5th. There is much legislation in the UK surrounding fireworks; the minimum age limit and restricted purchase periods certainly help reduce the mental anguish of pets, although it is presumably driven from the human safety angle as much as any other. It still remains, however, that in the UK, fireworks can be set off on any evening (before 11pm, but sometimes later), from any private garden and by any adult.

Maybe you love the bangs. That's fine, I don't want to stop them. I'm not a fan of restricting personal freedoms; but, as with smoking and drinking laws, when something affects others, I feel there has to be some give and take. Between 2018 and 2019, the NHS reported nearly 2,000 visitors to A&E in England and Wales on account of fireworks, and many ended up as hospital admissions. Also noted is that in firework season their advice webpage for burns and scalds suddenly spikes with visits, suggesting many more minor injuries occur that don't result in a trip to A&E. Other statistics show that the safest place to enjoy fireworks (other than following my example and staying indoors) is at an organised display. Home garden events and even sparklers result in a lot of injuries. As a vet and a pet owner, all I'm hoping for is that you'll now recognise that animals also suffer badly on account of fireworks.

Currently, it is considered courteous to inform your neighbours if you are setting off fireworks, but that only helps a little. The bangs can be heard from blocks away; are you going to leaflet-drop several hundred houses? With modern technology, a solution is simple. What about a system whereby all fireworks displays, from big shows to tiny private garden events, must be registered with the local council? All events could then be posted on a website to which people (I'm thinking pet owners) could subscribe for alerts when a new event is added, stating the date, time and postcode. Perhaps the ability to register an event might be tied in with the possession of a 'certificate of competence', acquired by way of a basic course on safety.

Diazepam, first marketed as Valium, is one of the prescription options for temporary relief of anxiety on Bonfire Night. It is an 'anxiolytic' – it helps calm animals down by relieving anxiety and often sedates them at the same time. But that isn't always the case. I tried it with Fyrish one night, in anticipation of the fireworks, and instead of 'chilling out', she went completely the other way and spent an hour or so 'wired to the moon'. Like a pantomime horse, she merrily romped around the house, but at least she didn't care a hoot about the fireworks!

Unfortunately, a variety of individual responses to certain medications can occur. The other classic incident I can remember with diazepam involved a cat that was brought to me with a complete loss of appetite. I was a young vet working as a locum on the Isle of Wight at the time. I could find no immediate reason for its inappetence and felt the important initial step was to get a meal into it. I knew that injecting diazepam into a cat's vein would, along with other possible effects such as sedation, have the very useful consequence of making it ravenously hungry for a few minutes. (It's worth adding that other medications are more often used in preference today.)

I dutifully administered the drug and placed a bowl of food in front of my patient, fully expecting to see the usual instant positive reaction, and admittedly feeling more than a little bit smug at how impressed the owner would be at my quick fix to her cat's problem. However, old Murphy and his law have been stalking me from a young age; much to the client's surprise, and my horror, the cat decided it wanted to be one of the minority that manifests a paradoxical reaction. Did it go woozy? Did it tuck into its food? No, it shot off around the surgery, which was unfortunately rather open-plan, like a hare on a racing track. I pursued it at greyhound speed, and after a chase scene more in keeping with a *Tom and Jerry* cartoon, it headed straight for an open window.

I ended up at the doctor for some antibiotics. It turned out the cat was hungry after all; as I narrowly prevented an embarrassing escape, it sank its teeth into my hand.

Chapter Twenty-Five

The Highland Seals

The solitude and peace of our coastline in winter offers more than just soul food for those of us who enjoy a brisk clifftop walk. The undisturbed beaches and interconnecting coves, bays and sheltered estuaries also provide an ideal nursery environment for the seal species of Scotland. Indeed, the quality of our inshore habitat is so great for these sleek swimmers that an estimated 30 per cent of the entire European seal population is believed to reside on Scottish shores.

Two species of seal bask, breed and feed in the waters around the Caithness coastline: the grey seal and the harbour seal. Given the long nights and the chances of some seriously foul and cold weather, you would think that winter would be a very poor choice for any wild animal to be giving birth. Yet, starting in the autumn and carrying through into winter, female grey seals haul themselves out onto our beaches and deliver their snowy-white fluff-covered pups.

Our seas are rich hunting grounds for seals, and the expectant grey seal mums are in fine fettle come the cooler months due to storing fat from a long summer of feeding on fish; so, perhaps it's not completely confounding as to why they choose this time to birth their young. The fluffy white fur of the newborn pups may simply be nothing more than a warm, cosy coat, but one hypothesis suggests that it could also be a protective camouflage from predators for those born onto ice, and might be a hangover from when ice cloaked a larger dome of the northern hemisphere. Still, the species thrives well today despite the fact that most, certainly here in Scotland, are born on ice-less beaches and rocks. In the water seals fall prey to sharks and orcas; on land perhaps only an occasional sea eagle is a threat to a pup – although, formerly, humans fit that bill too.

Seeing these vulnerable-looking seal pups alone on our beaches is not unusual in winter, but it helps to understand a little more of their biology before you jump to the conclusion that a lone pup is always in need of help. All mammalian mothers initially rear their young on milk, and seal milk is particularly high in fat. Grey seal pups can gorge on up to two and a half litres of milk daily and gain as much as 30kg in just the first two weeks from birth. The mother might lose twice that figure in body mass throughout this period of high demand before weaning, despite occasionally nipping off to forage in the sea, and returning to her pup after a bite to eat. When pups are only two to three weeks of age, milk feeding stops and the young must endure a period of fasting for a week or more before diving in to learn to fish for themselves. This strategy of intense feeding with high-energy milk followed by the mandate to 'find your own food' is common among seal species and means their lactation periods are some of the shortest of all mammals.

So, if you stumble across a lone seal pup, the chances are it is not sick or injured; although it may look hungry and abandoned, this could well be part of nature's plan. Don't be thrown by its tatty appearance. It's probably just a grey seal pup losing its white coat in preparation for its upcoming seafaring adventure. Unless you notice large sores and wounds, or that it's exceptionally unresponsive to your proximity, then human disturbance and intervention is not warranted. Indeed, the SSPCA warn that any well-meaning contact could even deter a seal mother from returning to her pup; you will have done more harm than good.

There are always going to be those inevitable, yet unfortunate, cases where a grey or harbour seal pup is not destined to make it to adulthood. In the wild, and nearly always away from our gaze, it is estimated that almost half of the seals born on our shores will die. If their mothers become sick or injured, or die at sea, then they are obviously going to be unable to feed their young. There are also cases where a mum will abandon a pup before it has made its optimum weight, not through illness, but down to poor maternal instinct. Sometimes, too, seal pups will become separated from their mothers in rough seas and storms. In such cases, you may well find a pup that is quite obviously weak and malnourished. Also, as with any particularly young animal, they are prone to illness and injury. Just making it to the point where they stand a chance of breeding for themselves has the odds of tossing a coin. As well as the predators mentioned, pups can be attacked and fatally wounded by other seals: as a species harbour seals are smaller than the greys, and the latter can bully the former. Grey males have even been found to attack pups of their own species.

In any case, if you find a seal that you reckon *does* justify the need for human intervention, the SSPCA advise that you *do not* approach it or try to return it to the water. Maintain a safe distance and call your appropriate national or local animal rescue charity for advice. In Caithness, it is the SSPCA or the BDMLR who bring in seals from the wild to us, and not members of the public.

This winter Jennifer and I discovered a grey seal pup while out walking along a local beach. I found myself in a slightly amusing situation, though. I was actually the vet on call that day, and was just having a brief stroll on my break between calls when we found the animal. I pondered: *If it is in genuine need of help, do I call the SSPCA, knowing that they would attend, find the poor chap but then call me right back to treat it?* I parked those thoughts for a few moments, and, in my capacity as vet, I felt justified in briefly getting closer than I would advise the public, in order to make my assessment of the animal without causing any undue distress.

It did have a little bit of its fluffy white coat left, but it was alert and in fair bodily condition with no obvious injuries. By the criteria already outlined, I determined it to be a case of 'leave it alone'. I called the SSPCA and listened to their very informative message while waiting for someone to answer. From the content of the message, it was apparent that calls about seals were not uncommon; so I hung up. But there were other walkers with dogs on the beach, so I opted to phone again anyway, just to fill them in, as they could well have received other calls raising concern about what might have been perceived to be an animal in need.

Seals have truly captured the heart of a nation. They are the poster-child species for so many marine conservation charities and are a big draw for nature-spotting tours around the Scottish Highlands and islands. It isn't hard to see why. With their large dark eyes, cute whiskers and apparently playful behaviours – bobbing around in the sea or lumbering around comically on land – they seem to elicit a cooing response from even the most steel-hearted human. However, for us vets, our reaction on hearing that a seal has been brought into the practice is very different.

'Seals,' to quote vet Shondie, 'can be little savages.' They are agile and powerful animals that can react surprisingly quickly when their personal space is invaded, and they are armed with a ferocious set of jaws and teeth. Getting bitten by one won't simply cause you a serious wound; they also carry some very dangerous bacteria in their mouths. This can bring on an infection known as 'seal finger', which was once fairly common among the seal-hunting peoples of Scandinavia and the Arctic Circle. It causes pain, redness, discharge and swelling and can even lead to joint infection. It wasn't until 1991 that the likely causative agent – a bacterium – was identified. Nowadays it can be treated with anti-biotics, but back in the commercial seal hunting heyday in the eighteenth and nineteenth centuries, you would be lucky to escape the infection without the need for amputation.

Although intrigued to tackle something new, I can remember feeling nervous about examining seals when I first came to Caithness, and I quizzed our senior vets in great depth about exactly the best methods for handling and treating them. Regardless of how cuddly these animals might look when comfortably doing their own thing, when you enter a pen to attempt an examination, they will change instantly: hissing out a warning first, then baring their teeth and poising to strike, all to ward off what is understandably perceived to be their assailant. With that in mind, it is fortunate for us that the seals that are brought to our practice are nearly always youngsters, but nevertheless, we take no chances. We wear gloves to lessen the chance of being contaminated by the seal's bacteria, and one person will distract the seal while another throws a towel over it from behind, before quickly pinning it with a thigh either side of its body and firmly gripping the back of its head. Once we have them in that position, they are usually fairly easy to examine and treat, as long as you remain on your guard. So far, none of our vets (not even Ken) has been bitten.

On examination, minor wounds and lacerations are common findings. These will have been picked up as part of the natural rough and tumble of a life at sea, but any significant ones may need to be treated. Often, the pups are just weak from exposure, dehydration and malnourishment as a result of abandonment. In such cases we will usually give them an electrolyte solution via a tube down the throat, and if required, we may also place them under a heat lamp for the night. If they have an infection or illness that we think will be helped by antibiotics, then we will administer them by injection, but we might also dispense tablets to be given over a few days.

Treating seal pups long-term is not something the practice is adequately set up to do. When they are brought to us, the longest they will ever stay is a night. Then they are taken to a specialist seal rehabilitation centre, usually the SSPCA's National Wildlife Rescue Centre, where they care for about 100 pups a year before releasing them back into the wild. Our job is to assess the extent of their illness or injury and then either begin the process of treatment or make them more comfortable before they are later taken for rehabilitation. As with other wildlife, we sadly must make the welfare decision to euthanise some seals if we believe they really won't make it.

One of the most bizarre seal jobs I have ever had to do came several years before *The Highland Vet* was filmed. It was actually the surgery's first brush with the world of television, with a major British TV channel, in fact. The production team called early one morning out of the blue; they wanted to fix a tracker to a large ocean-going seal for a children's programme so that viewers could follow it 'live' on a journey in and around the Atlantic. They had a vet with them but needed more sedative, so I offered our premises for the task and helped as best I could. The sedation was a bit of a challenge on an animal so large and unusual, and gluing the tracker to its back was quite a struggle. In the end, I don't know if it was a particularly successful experiment and I'm not entirely sure it was even broadcast. I later heard a rumour that instead of bleeping its way through hundreds of miles of ocean for the thrill of the young audience, the tracker was, allegedly, very soon picked up transmitting from a single stationary position somewhere deep down on the seabed.

On *The Highland Vet* series, as with many of our wildlife cases, we have featured that honest mix of the seals that pulled through and made it to the rehabilitation centre, and those that we had no option but to put to sleep. This year, though, the series did feature an uplifting seal story from one of our rarer species.

The harbour seal, also known as the common seal, is in fact a lot less common in our waters when compared to the grey seal. According to the Mammal Society, in British waters they number around 55,000 individuals, next to a population of some 120,000 grey seals. Furthermore, a recent study by NatureScot, the Scottish nature agency, records a decline in the number of harbour seals in the northern and eastern parts of our nation; it cites as potential causes possible exposure to toxins from harmful algae, predation by killer whales, and predation by and competition from grey seals. They are faring better to the west, but in our waters the harbour seal population is not as healthy as NatureScot would expect.

Harbour seals are particularly susceptible to being bullied away from feeding grounds, and even killed, by rival grey seals. Harbours can be distinguished from greys not only by their slighter size but also their blunter 'puppy face' and V-shaped nostrils. Their coats are spotty and variable in colour: they can be anything from a light brown through to a darker grey. And unlike the grey seal, their young are born during the summer, but a close encounter with this particular seal pup species in our practice is unusual at any time of the year.

Vet Ken was once tasked with dealing with a harbour seal on camera. It was estimated to be only four months old, and it topped the cuteness scale with its puppy-dog looks. This one sat innocently in one of our practice pens, looking like butter wouldn't melt in its mouth. Not only was it small but it had taken the characteristic dry-land posture of the harbour seal: lying down in an endearing banana shape, with its head and hind flippers elevated.

Ken was certainly not about to be fooled, though, and was fully aware of the risk any seal poses. Four months might seem very young – a near-helpless baby by our own standards – but harbour seal pups are exceptionally adept right from birth, and unlike greys, they will be swimming and diving at only a few hours old. This one could definitely already hunt fish, so biting a clumsy and naive vet wasn't going to present it with much of a challenge.

Ken explained to the camera that the seal had been spotted repeatedly coming into land by walkers at a couple of different beaches. It was suspected, then, that the wee lad had either lost his colony or been abandoned. Ken spotted a few wounds on the seal's body, some of which looked infected, and roped vet David in to help with a closer examination. 'They are very difficult to handle,' began Ken knowingly, while gazing at the bonny wee face in the pen. 'He might look pretty quiet and cute at the moment, but they are fast and extremely strong for their size.'

Ken had acquired a pile of towels to attempt to cover the seal and first tried dropping two smaller ones roughly on its head to cover its eyes. Both were easily and immediately pawed away with the seal's front flipper, like an expert boxer blocking a jab, so he next tried to smother it with a much larger one; but it somehow even managed to evade that and was soon scooting its way sharply along the concrete floor of the pen. 'Careful!' called Ken, as it attempted a somewhat futile escape beneath a set of metal shelves. As its head disappeared beneath the lower shelf, Ken clasped hold of its hind flippers and pulled it backwards for David to finally, and successfully, hurl the big towel right over its body and pin it to the floor. 'That wasn't the plan,' remarked David, while maintaining a firm grip on its head.

With Ken now able to get close enough to the animal, he could fully inspect its wounds. 'These guys are prone to being bullied by the big adults,' he surmised as he worked. 'Usually, on every beach there is a big, mean male that goes around attacking everybody that comes onto his patch.' This harbour seal had fallen victim to a larger seal, either one from its own colony or one of the notorious grey seals, and there was still pus leaking from his open wounds. Worse still, Ken's stethoscope revealed a crackling noise in the seal's chest, which indicated the likelihood of a lung infection.

'It's a bit frustrating,' said Ken. 'If it was just the wounds, I'd say release him, but we've got to make the best decision for his welfare. I'm concerned about his breathing, and if we release him back into the wild as he is, there is a really good chance that he'll just get preyed on again by another big seal.'

It's never an easy decision to make, but in this seal's case, Ken reasoned it would have a better chance of recovery if it was first given some time at the SSPCA sanctuary down in Inverness. To help it on its way, though, Ken tubed some electrolyte solution into it, replacing deficient fluids that it would normally have extracted from fish caught in the wild, before the SSPCA arrived to take it on the long journey down south.

As a vet's experience with wildlife grows, they learn to adopt a philosophical approach to the various cases that come through the door. With seals, they either don't make it out of our practice or are taken to a distant SSPCA rehabilitation centre, after which we rarely hear about them again. This little harbour seal was unusual, though. Before the planned journey to Inverness, it was first taken to our local SSPCA centre, where it made an unexpected over-night improvement. In fact, it was observed that the more it was just left alone, the more its breathing and general demeanour bounced back. After only one night at the surgery, and one night at the centre, it was returned to us for a final antibiotic injection to help its chest and the infected wounds. It was then decided that it was best to end intervention and added stress from the human species: the seal was to be taken home to the rocky shores and chilly seawater of the Pentland Firth.

At the harbour in Brough, just east of Dunnet Head, the pup was released at a spot close to a known colony of harbour seals and was soon seen to be keenly working his way across the exposed tangle of kelp and back out to sea.

We rarely know what happens next in the life of any wild animal after release, but, as with so many of our cases, beyond our medical treatment and best endeavours, we always retain a little hope; and that little seal's future was certainly a whole lot more hopeful than it had been just a couple of days previously.

Chapter Twenty-Six

The Not-So-Fine Art of Wrestling Pigs

Little mention has so far been made of a common farm species: the pig. I will try to address that omission now. We have relatively few pigs up here, but our intermittent encounters with them can most definitely stick in the mind. The biggest problem, I find, is their lack of 'handles'. The absence of a conventional neck that narrows behind the head means a halter or collar of any kind will not easily stay in place, even if you could get close enough to attach it. Harnesses are available, but unless you wish to leave one on every pig permanently, then you still have to manage to apply them in the first place. So, restraining a pig has its challenges. A snout rope could be used, plus there are ways and means of getting close to them by cornering them with a large board; but, as a rule, pigs are slippery characters and deafen anyone trying to do anything they perceive as even mildly threatening with their grunts and squeals. To exemplify this, I have two tales.

The first is recalled by vet Eilidh. A couple of years ago, she paid a visit to a kunekune. Historically, such pigs were kept by the New Zealand Maoris for meat, but this one in the northern hemisphere wasn't destined for the Christmas pigs in blankets; it was simply a pet.

The pig – let's call him Berty – had been treated recently by other vets, so he had become suspicious of strangers wafting syringes outside his cosy pigpen. He had a foot condition that now required a closer look and appropriate treatment. The problem Eilidh encountered was Berty's reluctance to leave the seclusion of his safe haven. For a full 20 minutes, she and Berty's owners attempted to coax him out with all sorts of treats, but he was too wise and wary. With a vet in view, not even his favourite titbits were enough of an enticement.

Thinking laterally, as vets often have to, Eilidh ultimately climbed onto the roof of the pen and hid from view while Berty's owners persuaded the wilful occupant out with a banana. Duped, the pig left his shelter for this choicest of snacks. Eilidh then sprang into action, leapt off the pen and pounced from behind, voiding the contents of her sedative-filled syringe into Berty's backside before he knew what had happened. At the same time, the entrance to the pen was blocked. The porcine patient soon entered a semi-sedated state, allowing Eilidh to perform the tasks required.

My second short, curly tale begins with a call to a large farm building where two young pigs had free roam of the whole space. The complaint was that one appeared to have suddenly gone blind, and once I'd assessed it, I had to agree. Top of my list was to rule out lead poisoning. Old vehicle batteries, lead pipes and paint could all be possible sources of this toxic metal for inquisitive pigs, but I struggled to find evidence of any of these in the building and the pig was relatively bright in other respects.

Apart from my wish to help my patient, lead residues in the body would render its meat a big health risk for any human consuming it. I suggested a blood test for lead levels and told the pig keeper I would call back later to draw samples (I don't remember why now – perhaps I didn't have the right equipment). He said he wouldn't be available to assist later, but I felt confident that I would manage with just a few minutes' help from another vet.

No guessing is required as to whom that vet might have been. Of course, Ken drew the short straw and ended up roped in to form a double act with me for another veterinary pantomime. It was the middle of winter and so, by our return late in the afternoon, it was already dark. Such a call wouldn't have been any fun without additional obstacles to add to our adventure: the building had no lighting. But fear not! Ken had his trusty head torch and I had a flashlight. Anyway, how hard could it be? The blind pig couldn't see us coming!

We entered the building and found the pigs snoozing on a pile of hay. I planned to hit an ear vein with my needle; it would be the most accessible option, provided the pig stayed still for a few moments. With his head torch illuminating his path, Ken stealthily crept up on his prey from behind and pinned it between his thighs – much as we do for seals. It squealed and squirmed, and I started to grapple with its ear.

But remember? No handles! The pig shot out of Ken's grip and around the building – blindness not seeming to be a worry for it at all – and Ken landed on his behind. We pursued it briefly but both realised this was only going to end in two tired vets, two stressed pigs and a heap more embarrassment than we'd already experienced. I had to inform the owner I'd be back for a third time the next morning.

I returned in daylight, restrained the pig using boards, and, through a small gate to allow access, managed to retrieve a blood sample from its neck with minimal fuss. After all that, the laboratory found no evidence of lead poisoning, and the pig regained its sight without further vet involvement. Hardly a Christmas miracle; I considered other possible diagnoses such as salt poisoning or dehydration. In the end, though, it was a hard-earned reminder that sometimes nature can resolve problems on its own in spite of our best efforts as vets.

Chapter Twenty-Seven

The Worst Christmas Pudding of All Time

Apart from the expected celebrations – the Christmas lights being switched on in town, the festive market, seasonal window displays and the community carol services – for a vet in Caithness, December also brings the staff Christmas party and vomit. Not that those two are necessarily linked; I'm really thinking more about dogs in this instance.

As you know from the antics described in summer, the eating of undesirable items and substances is a common reason for dogs to be presented at the veterinary clinic. Dogs have a good vomit reflex; it could be considered a compensatory mechanism for a relatively undiscerning palate. *I don't know what it is, but it smells pungent. Therefore I must eat it quickly before my owner catches me.* They rely on the fallback that anything that can't be processed will be rejected by the act of vomiting. However, despite dogs getting away with such dietary indiscretion the majority of the time, on occasion whatever putrid item one has eaten manages to introduce enough turmoil or infection into the digestive system to cause a bout of persistent vomiting and diarrhoea and warrant a trip to the vet. In severe cases, this may even necessitate hospitalisation.

On other occasions, evidence of scattered wrappers and packaging leaves the owner in little doubt that an offence has been perpetrated, and yet the substances eaten are unlikely to elicit natural vomiting because they are designed to be ingested and are intended to stay down. Medications are an obvious example. Dogs will often manage to find their owner's medicine supply and tuck into it. A frantic phone call ensues whereby we look up the drug's details and, with an estimate of how much may have been consumed, we make a judgement as to whether 'induced emesis' is required. By that I mean we administer something that deliberately makes an animal vomit.

The other classic situation is the consumption of chocolate. In the run-up to Christmas, in many guises such as selection boxes, a seemingly innocent threat is lurking in larger quantities than usual around people's homes. Sometimes it is right under the family pet's nose around the Christmas tree. We mustn't forget (although it seems we sometimes do) that dogs are used professionally by police and other agencies to detect traces of explosives or narcotics; sniffing chocolate through a bit of Christmas wrapping is not a tall order.

I recall, from time to time, consuming far too much chocolate as a child on Christmas Day. I would feel over-full and wish my eyes hadn't been bigger than my belly, but that was all – no panic and no rush to hospital. Yet for a dog, such overindulgence could have very serious consequences. Dogs are particularly sensitive to the caffeine-like chemical called theobromine that is present in cocoa beans. Theobromine exerts many effects within the canine body: it is a general stimulant, causing hyperexcitability and possible fits, and it makes the heart race and develop abnormal rhythms. Due to their peculiar sensitivity, overdose can occur in dogs after eating a portion considered small by a human. This could result in admission for intensive treatment, and may very occasionally prove fatal. In particular, cocoa powder and dark chocolate are loaded with this dangerous substance, and a small dog wouldn't need to swallow a lot to put its life at risk. Even a Labrador munching on a medium to large bar of dark choco-late could endanger itself. Smaller portions may be safe, and milk chocolate contains a lower proportion of theobromine, so larger quantities of it can be tolerated; the dose needs to be considered relative to the dog's body weight.

'Chocolate calculators' are available online for vets, or indeed anyone, to use. Enter the dog's weight with the estimated weight of chocolate eaten, and whether it was dark or milk, and you can get an idea as to whether a risky dose has been ingested. If the result is in the red, we need to make the dog vomit as soon as possible. If in the green, then there is little risk other than perhaps a minor gut upset.

Theobromine affects human bodies too. Some people may have learnt that they need to be sparing with their chocolate consumption, but in general, as a species, we are not overly sensi-tive like our canine companions. Just so you can continue to indulge without fear, any sensible person would feel bloated and sick long before they had managed to ingest enough chocolate to risk experiencing the dangerous effects of the theobromine it contained. Despite that good news, you may never want to eat chocolate again after the next story.

By far the most notorious offenders that I have come across in regard to eating household items and substances were Alfie and Momo. These two beagles belonged to Martha, a friend of mine from church, who is the epitome of a nice-but-nutty dog lover. Every vet's surgery in the country will have a Martha or two on their books; her life is her dogs, and a friendship external to the vet-client relationship seems superfluous on account of seeing her so regularly at the clinic. Not only did the pair of beagles seem to be the most unfortunate dogs in relation to disease and injury, but it feels that they have been made to vomit more times than I've held down hot dinners. Vets use a drug called apomorphine to induce vomiting in dogs, and because of Martha's two partners in crime, I wonder whether the board of the pharmaceutical company took home extra Christmas bonuses for several years. Regular vet visits to eject the contents of their stomachs occurred throughout the beagles' colourful lives.

A fear of any parent is that their children will become associated with kids considered to be bad influences. A friend often walked our own dog Milis while Jennifer and I were out at work and, as she was also friends with Martha, they would often arrange to meet up and explore the Highland countryside together with all three dogs. One such day, when Milis was a young and impressionable Labrador, I received a phone call while on lunch. A colleague at the clinic had been presented with Alfie and Momo, who had gone missing on a walk for a prolonged period and, when eventually found, were merrily bloated and coated with stinky green stuff around their jowls. They had found a deer carcass in the woods and had munched on it with gusto. My colleague assessed the risk and, due to the potential for bowel blockage or gastroenteritis given the decomposed nature of the feast, it was decided to clear them out using the faithful (and by now familiar) apomorphine injection. I was asked for permission to do the same to Milis, who had disappeared with them on this occasion and had telltale signs that she might have been participating in the same gory gluttony; of course, the sensible thing was for me to say yes. To this day I maintain her innocence; Milis was led astray by a couple of rogues and would not have been hanging her head in shame before one of my colleagues had she been out walking without the pack.

Beagles are renowned for their nose. One memorable December evening, I was on call and the phone summoned me with its familiar foreboding tone. It was Martha. Perhaps it was church business, I thought optimistically. But no, it soon became apparent that yet another saga involving her dogs was unfolding. I was informed that the bothersome beagles had gained access to a huge cache of chocolate purchased as Christmas gifts for nephews and nieces. I don't even think we bothered with a chocolate calculator. I just said, 'Get them to the surgery straight away.'

For obvious reasons, I often use a corner of the car park as my consulting room when asking a dog to empty its stomach. So, there we were: Martha, Alfie, Momo and me, on a cold, dark December evening, gathered around a drain and awaiting the inevitable effect of the apomorphine injection. Alfie, in particular, looked rotund compared to his usual self and so I knew we were doing the right thing.

A few minutes after an injection, as apomorphine takes effect, slight sedation becomes apparent and then an expression of apprehension follows as the dog starts to feel queasy. Alfie was first to make his offering. An enormous portion of chocolate pudding was served up, although it would have won no prizes for presentation on *MasterChef*. Then Momo – a similar offering. Then more, then more, then more …

Apomorphine often creates two or three waves of vomiting, each wave comprising three or four evacuations. After clearing their stomachs, by wave number two or three dogs are often dry-retching, and owner and vet alike are wishing there was a counter-injection to turn it off. Is it possibly a bit harsh to say, 'Serves them right'? The beagles continued to produce chocolate well into wave two. The sheer overall quantity of molten chocolate produced that evening was astounding. The first few piles were huge, followed by smaller piles of, let's say, chocolate mousse, on account of the mélange of foamy saliva and gastric mucus. I had never seen such a yield from induced emesis.

Although deliberately standing to watch dogs vomit is not likely to be a common social activity, there is normally time to make small talk for a quarter of an hour before the apomorphine's effect starts to wane; I've shared some interesting conversations in this time over the years with a variety of individuals. That evening Martha explained that she knew what her dogs were like and so had secured the chocolate up high in a closed cupboard. The dastardly duo had sniffed it out, broken into the cupboard, tumbled the stash to the ground and devoured it all, with much of the wrapping included. Martha was then faced with the prospect of buying more Christmas gifts for her nephews and nieces and finding a beagle-proof facility to store them in.

We waited until it seemed no further vomiting would follow and then the three of them sheepishly left for home. The beagles had eaten mainly milk chocolate, but as I cleared away the multiple sickly-sweet mounds and hosed down the car park, I concluded that they had consumed easily enough to make themselves very ill, if not put their lives at risk.

Chapter Twenty-Eight

The Year Ends at Thurso

As the year draws to a close, it is customary to reflect on things gone by – the good, the bad and the ugly – to say farewell to the water under the bridge and to look forward with anticipation to whatever the future may hold.

The circle of life, which is a phrase I'm unable to say without starting to sing a certain song from *The Lion King*, will continue to cycle onward, here in the far north of Scotland as on the plains of Africa. The new year will once more bring new life as those early lambs herald the coming rush of spring. The farming calendar has flowed from calving to turnout, from silage-making to harvest, and from the arrival of newborns through to livestock sales. The days have changed from short and cold to long and warm, and now back again. The Highland vets have, quite literally, had their hands in creation's drama as it has played out across the fields and farms of Caithness and north Sutherland, and those same hillsides and homesteads now cry 'Encore!' as the new year beckons.

On a wider timescale, this notion of the circle of life was brought home to me rather poignantly this year on Christmas

Eve. As others were cosying up, hanging their stockings and watching Christmas classics on TV, one couple were suffering the emotional trauma of seeing the circle finally close for one of their beloved dogs. They phoned the practice to ask if they could bring in their old bearded collie; his health had suddenly deteriorated and the time had come for me to facilitate a peaceful and dignified departure.

I sedated the poor old chap before the final injection, and as he began to doze in the owner's lap, her husband commented how it had all disappeared in the twinkling of an eye. 'I remember, it was you, Guy, who gave him his first check-over and vaccines as a puppy. It seems like yesterday.' He paused to take in the sobering reality of his comment and then offered, 'You've been here a while now, haven't you?'

I nodded and quipped, 'Indeed, some of us vets used to be young puppies, but now we're turning into old dogs!'

But let's be reasonable. I like to think there's still some life in this old dog; I'm only in my early fifties. Yet, one day when I do eventually hang up my stethoscope and lay down my scalpel for good, the circle of life in general practice must continue for the sake of all the farm stock, horses, pets and wildlife casualties out there. I see the young vets quickly learning the ropes, rapidly increasing in competence, and I know that the care of this area's animals will remain in good hands. I wonder what new gadgets will one day revolutionise their working lives, and what new expectations will inspire their dedication and drive for excellence. I am confident, though, that whether TV cameras follow them or not, the Highland vets will always have a vital role in the community up here.

On Christmas Day, once my on-call shift was over, we drove a couple of hours southwards within the Highland region to spend time with my wife's extended family. On our return to the far north the next day, as we approached the Causeway Mire, I recognised a familiar face in a four-by-four pickup truck pulling off the road ahead. I stopped alongside and wound down my window.

Farmer James smiled back at us. For his veterinary needs, he uses the Wick branch of our practice and so I have never personally touched any of his cows, but Jennifer and I became friendly with James and Moira, his wife, while our children and theirs competed against each other, or performed alongside each other, at local musical events over the years.

For Jennifer and me, this was our first Christmas with no children at home, as they move on to forge the next part of the circle in their own lives. We shared news with James and contemplated the passage of time before setting out on the final leg of our journey across the great Causeway Mire.

The encounter with a familiar face brought the realisation that the barely inhabited expanse of the Flow Country stretching out before me was now also in itself a very familiar face – that of my home territory. On a clear December afternoon, staring across miles of open terrain to the mountains beyond, I found this vast tract of land no longer held the same sense of eerie desolation as it had the first time I'd traversed it, on the day of my job interview nearly two and a half decades ago. I guess it hasn't done so for a while. Now it was welcoming me with open arms, beckoning me home across its ancient blanket of peat to the small town of Thurso.

Acknowledgements

There will always be so many people to thank in relation to a work such as this. My wife, Jennifer, has watched me obsess and pore over these pages for months and tolerated uncomplainingly my inattention to her, whilst offering a few welcome gems of wisdom as the drafts were read. Daisybeck Studios is certainly deserving of a mention. This television production company saw something in our veterinary practice and its team which we hadn't appreciated for ourselves. They trusted that the great British public would be interested in our daily work and the magnificent area that surrounds us, and from that exposure in the series *The Highland Vet* came the opportunity to author a book; an experience which has been preoccupying and yet very rewarding. I wish to thank Will Millard for laughing heartily at my anecdotes and for all his enthusiastic help in bringing this work to fruition. Of course, gratitude goes to my editors Claire Collins and Jessica Anderson for their insightful comments and grammatical fixes. The generations either side of me should also be acknowledged. Firstly, my children for coping with a father who frequently smelled and who so often disappeared after the phone rang. Moreover, without the support of my parents I would never have made it into and through vet school and had the opportunity to forge a career, the stories from which hopefully provided some interest to those who have thumbed these pages. But the book is far greater than one person. The biggest thank you must go to my colleagues, our clients and the animals of this region, without whom these pages would have been few and their content lifeless.